Ethical Issues and the Religious and Historical Basis for the Objection of Jehovah's Witnesses to Blood Transfusion Therapy

Ethical Issues and the Religious and Historical Basis for the Objection of Jehovah's Witnesses to Blood Transfusion Therapy

André Carbonneau

Studies in Religion and Society
Volume 63

The Edwin Mellen Press
Lewiston•Queenston•Lampeter

Library of Congress Cataloging-in-Publication Data

Carbonneau, André.
Ethical issues and the religious and historical basis for the objection of Jehovah's Witnesses to blood transfusion therapy / André Carbonneau
p. cm. -- (Studies in religion and society ; v. 63)
Includes bibliographical references and index.
ISBN 0-7734-6542-1
1. Jehovah's Witnesses--Controversial literature. 2. Blood--Transfusion--Religious aspects--Jehovah's Witnesses. 3. Blood--Transfusion--Moral and ethical aspects. I. Title. II. Studies in religion and society (New York, N.Y.) ; v. 63.

BX8526.5.C37 2004

2003044260

This is volume 63 in the continuing series
Studies in Religion and Society
Volume 63 ISBN 0-7734-6542-1
SRS Series ISBN 0-88946-863-X

A CIP catalog record for this book is available from the British Library.

The Edwin Mellen Press
Box 450
Lewiston, New York
USA 14092-0450

The Edwin Mellen Press
Box 67
Queenston, Ontario
CANADA L0S 1L0

The Edwin Mellen Press, Ltd.
Lampeter, Ceredigion, Wales
UNITED KINGDOM SA48 8LT

Printed in the United States of America

To my loving wife Mary for her continued support and assistance

CONTENTS

Preface

By

Mark Boyd, MD, FRCSC, FRCOG, FACOG

I was happy to be asked to write a preface for this book. The issues that are dealt with in the text are important both to the general public and to the medical community. The author, André Carbonneau, is a distinguished lawyer who has special expertise in bioethics. He has applied this knowledge to explore, in a very close way, the relationship between physician and patient. He is specifically concerned with a patient's right to accept or refuse medical treatment.

A number of years ago the relationship between a physician and his patient was often paternalistic. The physician took the viewpoint that he himself was the one who was best suited to determine what was best for the patient. In other words the individual adult was treated as a dependent child. No one would argue in favor of such an attitude today.

The paternalistic approach was replaced by the doctrine of informed consent. In this process the physician gives medical information to the patient; he explains both the benefits and risks of the proposed treatment; after thoughtful discussion the patient either accepts or refuses the proffered medical advice. The physician or surgeon will only proceed with the recommended treatment with the patient's permission.

In a general sort of way the medical and legal community has had no difficulty in accepting the doctrine of informed consent when the patient refuses treatment on medical grounds. As example, it is an everyday experience for a patient to refuse, for a variety of reasons, chemotherapy or radical surgery for treatment of a life threatening cancer. In my experience the caregivers are understanding and supportive of the patient's difficult decision, even if they may not agree with it.

Crises may arrive, however, when patients refuse medical treatment for religious or moral reasons. These patients have been given the appropriate medical information but they have come to the conclusion that their religious or moral objections are of overriding importance. The medical community is often unable to understand or accept the patient's right to refuse medical treatment for such reasons, and his or her autonomy and right of self-determination are often questioned. Traditional rules often seem to be insufficient, forgotten or not applicable.

Clearly this is an important issue and important principles are involved. Given Mr Carbonneau's legal training it is understandable that he chooses to illustrate the issues and principles by means of a case study. This particular case study is that of the refusal of Jehovah's Witnesses patients to accept blood products. It is an apt and logical subject for study, for we have a large group of patients, with a clearly defined belief, who are against a frequently proposed medical treatment. This is a serious issue. Mr Carbonneau details the basis for Jehovah's Witnesses' beliefs, and by doing so lets us understand the depth of their commitment and to the fact that their refusal of blood products is a central principle of their religion. There is a legal saying that the "law is not concerned with small things." Certainly Mr Carbonneau is not discussing a small or in any way an unimportant issue.

As a medical doctor I especially profited from reading the history of blood usage in medical practice. The author shows that in ancient times mythical properties were given to blood. It was only in the 20th century that physicians stopped "bleeding" patients of large quantities of blood for many different ailments. The change and the popularity of the reverse practice, namely blood transfusion, came as a result of the relatively recent experience of military surgeons. The unrestricted usage of blood and the ensuing tragedies that we are all too familiar with are detailed. Mr Carbonneau certainly gives a positive note showing that alternatives to blood transfusion are available and effective and are becoming an increasingly important part of current medical practice.

Jehovah's Witnesses have been the driving force for the development of "non-blood medical and surgical management." There is no question that their efforts in that regard have been beneficial to both Witness and non-Witness patients. In a similar way, it should not be forgotten that Jehovah's Witnesses' legal battles for the rights of patients to refuse unwanted medical treatment has increased the civic liberties of everyone. This text allows us to better appreciate what has been done in this regard.

The author has shown that the physician who is "informed" as to his or her patients' beliefs and values "will serve his patients well, in keeping with fundamental legal and ethical issues." I believe that Mr Carbonneau has also served both his own and a much wider community by undertaking this work. It has been especially well done. Congratulations and many thanks!!

INTRODUCTION:

THE 'INFORMED DOCTOR'

The medical profession has long struggled with the concept of competent patients making final decisions regarding treatment. While in most developed countries courts have recognized and protected the right of patients to make such decisions, those refusing a particular medical treatment for non-medical reasons are viewed with suspicion. This is often the case when standard medical treatment is refused because of religious beliefs or for moral considerations. Even though their refusal of a particular treatment does not mean a refusal of all other medical treatments, and alternative treatment will probably be requested, patients taking such a stand are still viewed by many as seeking an early death.

Informed consent, a concept that developed in the twentieth century, is the rule applied to the doctor-patient relationship allowing the doctor to proceed with a recommended treatment. When obtaining informed consent from a patient, emphasis is placed on relevant medical information and on the risks and benefits of the proposed treatment. This concept, however, does not address the situation where medical treatment is refused for *non-medical* reasons. In such situations, the success of the doctor-patient relationship will largely depend on the doctor being well informed and understanding the reasons for the patient's refusal.

A case in point is that of Jehovah's Witnesses. Their refusal of blood transfusion (whole blood, red cells, white cells, platelets, or blood plasma) is well known, but often misunderstood.

While it is true that different religious groups may object, for various reasons, to certain medical treatments or procedures, Jehovah's Witnesses have been chosen as a case study because of the extensive worldwide[1] attention that they have received both in medical and legal journals.[2] Since blood transfusion therapy is a standard medical procedure, the Witnesses' objection to this particular treatment presents an ethical and legal challenge for medical communities in nearly all major countries.[3]

What is the religious basis for their belief? What efforts are being made to inform and help the medical community understand the nature of their refusal? If blood is forced upon a Witness patient, what are the consequences? Are the life-saving properties of blood exaggerated? Do alternative treatments really work?

The answers to these and other questions, in the light of ethical and legal guidelines, will help to determine the following: What guidelines should apply when a patient, deemed to be in a life-and-death situation, chooses, for religious or moral reasons, alternative treatment which may seem less efficient, or no treatment at all?

While obtaining the *informed consent of patients* in these circumstances is of primary importance, the 'informed doctor' approach, where the doctor is well informed and understands the underpinning of the patient's medical treatment decision, may be just as important, if not more.

---

[1] According to the 2003 Yearbook of Jehovah's Witnesses (p. 31) in 2002, there was a maximum of 6,304,645 Witnesses in 234 lands worldwide.

[2] For example, a search via the Internet in 45 medical journals from 1966-1999 on the website "MDConsult.com" produced 2911 articles referring to medical, ethical and legal issues raised by the refusal of allogeneic blood transfusion by Jehovah's Witnesses.

[3] However, recent scandals involving contaminated blood have caused both the government and the medical profession to reevaluate issues arising from blood transfusion therapy. See Krever, "Interim Report" as well as "Proceedings and Recommendations from the Symposium," Building a Blood System for the 21st century, held on 3-4 November 1997 in Toronto.

Section 1
JEHOVAH'S WITNESSES AND BLOOD TRANSFUSION

1. The Basis for Their Objection to Blood Transfusion

While different religious groups have their particular reasons for objecting to certain forms of medical treatment,[4] Jehovah's Witnesses are unique in their consistent and adamant objection to blood transfusion. To deal effectively with this situation, the treating physician must first of all comprehend the theological basis for their belief, not with a view to agreeing or disagreeing, but for the sole purpose of understanding the importance they attach to this doctrine.

Jehovah's Witnesses believe that God forbids humans from consuming human or animal blood under any circumstances. They believe this divine commandment to apply to any form of consumption, whether it be the ingestion of blood or its absorption through intravenous means. Hence, they request medical alternatives to blood transfusion therapy. As stated in one of their publications addressed to the medical profession and produced to assist their members when in a hospital setting: "They highly value life, and they seek good medical care. But they are determined not to violate God's standard, which has been consistent: Those who respect life as a gift from the Creator do not try to sustain life by taking in blood."[5]

---

[4] Manners, "When religious faith dictates treatment," 16; Lammers, "Dealing with other cultures and religions emphasized at recent ethics conference," 1211; Atighetchi, "Bioethics and Islam," 26; Howe, "Influencing a patient's religious beliefs: mandate or no-man's land?" 194; See also Stevenson, "Refusing measles vaccine may put others at risk: study," A12. (This article refers to Canadian provinces that allow exemption from mandatory vaccinations on religious or philosophical grounds.) See also Macklin, "Ethical Relativism in a Multicultural Society," 1 for a description of cultural and religious issues in health care.

[5] How Can Blood Save Your Life?, 6.

Jehovah's Witnesses take this belief very seriously. It is fundamental to their faith. They believe that, since the Creator has given the gift of life to all living creatures, to respect God's teaching regarding the consumption of blood, is to respect the sacredness of life itself. To consume blood, either orally or through a transfusion, is a rejection of their Creator's law, thereby incurring his disapproval. Their everlasting life and happiness is at stake. They do not hesitate to obtain other medical assistance. They aggressively seek alternative treatment to blood transfusion and have gone to great lengths to support their members in their effort to abide by what they perceive to be God's standard on blood.

Theological reasons for their refusal of blood

Jehovah's Witnesses refer to the Bible[6] to support their belief that it is forbidden for humans to consume human or animal blood, either by eating or through transfusions. They hold the Bible to be God's word revealing His purposes and standards to humankind.[7] Basic to their faith is the belief that abiding by God's Word, as they understand it, is necessary to obtain His approval and gain everlasting salvation, even when temporal life is threatened. It is also their view that God's laws, including the restriction on the use of blood, were given for the good of humankind. The observation of these laws will contribute to a measure of good health and happiness, even in a world that is less than perfect.[8] Thus, the health risks associated with blood transfusion therapy, highlighted in

---

[6] Unless otherwise indicated, all references from the Bible will be from the New International Version of The Holy Bible.

[7] On the question of whether the Bible is God's Word, see their publication: The Bible, God's Word or Man's?

[8] According to their publication Knowledge That Leads to Everlasting Life, 11: "Life's deepest and most disturbing questions are answered in the Bible. Accepting its guidance will help you to develop a friendship with God. What a grand privilege! And this will enable you to enjoy the peace that God alone can give," 21: "(...) when we read the Scriptures and apply their counsel, we are exercising wisdom that humans cannot achieve on their own, for the Bible is the book that reveals the knowledge of God that leads to everlasting life" and 217: "So you know that it is in your *lasting* best interest to serve God."

recent scandals involving tainted blood, is seen as a vindication of God's prohibition pertaining to the consumption of blood.[9]

Witnesses explain that the prohibition on the use of blood first appeared immediately after the Flood recorded in the Bible book of Genesis 9:3-6. According to this Biblical reference in which humans were officially[10] authorized to eat animal flesh, a specific commandment[11] regarding the blood of animals was given by God to Noah: "Everything that lives and moves will be food for you. … But you must not eat meat that has its lifeblood still in it."

Although authorized by God to eat the flesh of animals, Noah and his family were, however, forbidden to consume their blood.[12] Jehovah's Witnesses understand this commandment to apply not only to Noah and his family, but also to their descendants.[13] They support this belief by pointing to different occurrences throughout history when this same prohibition was repeated. For example, several centuries after the Flood, when Moses outlined God's Law Code to the ancient nation of Israel, he repeated the prohibition with regards to blood. Leviticus 17:10 states: "Any Israelite or any alien living among them who eats any blood – I will set my face against that person who eats blood and will cut him off from his people."[14]

---

9 See "Canada's 'Tainted Blood' Inquiry," Awake!, 20.

10 Some authors were of the view that animal flesh was already being consumed before the flood. For example, F. Delitzsch states: "Certainly men had already eaten not merely vegetable food and milk, but flesh also; this they had done however arbitrarily, they are now authorized to do it by Divine announcement." Delitzsch, A New Commentary on Genesis, 283.

11 Regarding this specific commandment, Adam Clarke wrote: "After the deluge it was prohibited, as we find above; and, being one of the *seven* Noahic precepts, it was not eaten previously to the Mosaic law. (…) This command is still scrupulously obeyed by the oriental Christians, and by the whole Greek Church; and why? Because the reasons still subsist." Clark, The Holy Bible, Containing the Old and New Testaments, 78.

12 Hastings, Dictionary of the Bible, 110: "Therefore though animals may be slaughtered for human food by the Noachic covenant (Genesis 9:1-7) the blood is not to be consumed; where the slaughter is at the altar, the blood goes to God at the altar; otherwise it is poured out."

13 They are not alone to hold this view, see *infra* endnotes 32, 33 and 34, and accompanying text.

14 This same prohibition on eating blood is repeated several times in ancient Israel's law. See for example the Bible book of Leviticus 7:26, 27 and the book of Deuteronomy 12:15, 16, 23-25, 27; 15:23.

In ancient Israel, slaughtered animals had to be bled if they were to be eaten. In the Law that he transmitted to the Israelites, Moses gave clear instructions to hunters as to what they were to do with the blood of animals. It was not to be consumed. According to Leviticus 17:13, 14: "Any Israelite or any alien living among you who hunts any animal or bird that may be eaten must drain out the blood and cover it with earth, because the life of every creature is its blood. That is why I have said to the Israelites, "You must not eat the blood of any creature, because the life of every creature is its blood."

All the law required was that the blood of the animal be drained. Jehovah's Witnesses take the view that this is in harmony with the command given to Noah. They do not, however, believe that the command "(Y)ou must not eat meat that has its lifeblood still in it." (Genesis 9:4) means that not a single particle of blood must remain in the slaughtered animal. "It was not required that the meat be squeezed or that it be soaked; simply that the blood be poured out."[15]

In Biblical times, Israelites were bound to observe this law, known as the Mosaic Law, as a fundamental part of their obedience to God. According to M'Clintock and Strong, this injunction applied to Israelites as well as to non-Israelites residing amongst them. The penalty for violating the law was "the being 'cut off from the people,' by which the punishment of death appears to be intended."[16]

Referring to the Bible, Witnesses explain the main reason for this prohibition: God attached a special meaning to blood — it represented life which he grants to all living beings, "for the life of all flesh is its blood."[17] They explain

---

[15] See "Questions From Readers," The Watchtower (1 November 1961), 670.

[16] "This strict injunction not only applied to the Israelites, but even to the strangers residing among them. The penalty assigned to its transgression was the being 'cut off from the people' by which the punishment of death appears to be intended (compare Hebrews 10:28), although it is difficult to ascertain whether it was inflicted by the sword or by stoning." McClintock and Strong's Cyclopoedia, 1:834.

[17] Leviticus 17:14.

that: "Blood had a symbolic meaning. It stood for life provided by the Creator. By treating blood as special, the people showed dependence on him for life. Yet, the main reason why they were not to take in blood was not that it was unhealthy, but that it had special meaning to God."[18]

The Bible ascribes to blood "the mysterious sacredness which belongs to life,"[19] whether animal or human. Thus, life, represented by blood, is sacred. This is illustrated by God's words to Cain after he murdered his brother Abel: "Your brother's blood cries out to me from the ground."[20] The pouring out of human blood did not go unnoticed by God, since it meant the loss of a life, and would eventually be formally prohibited.[21] Andrew Fuller (English Baptist minister and theologian, 1754-1815) also argues: "blood is the *life*, and God seems to claim it as sacred to himself."[22]

The Israelites of Bible times worshiped the same God as Noah and were also to consider blood as sacred. They were authorized to use it only in conjunction with worship to God, for atonement. Leviticus 17:11, 12 states: "For the life of a creature is in the blood, and I have given it to you to make atonement for yourselves on the altar; it is the blood that makes atonement for one's life. Therefore I say to the Israelites, 'None of you may eat blood, nor may an alien living among you eat blood.'"

While Jehovah's Witnesses do not believe that they are subject to the Mosaic Law,[23] they point to the prohibition on the consumption of blood in that

---

[18] How Can Blood Save Your Life? *supra* note 5, 4; See also Delitzsch, *supra* note 10, 284: "(A) sacred reverence for that principle of life flowing in the blood, which even as that of the animal is derived from God, who bestows a participation in His all-animating life."

[19] Smith, A Dictionary of the Bible, 94; See also Driver, The Book of Genesis, 96.

[20] Genesis 4:10.

[21] Among the laws Noah received, was the following: "Whoever sheds the blood of man, by man shall his blood be shed; for in the image of God has God made man." (Genesis 9:6).

[22] Fuller, Complete Works of the Rev. Andrew Fuller, with a Memoir of his life, 363.

[23] See You Can Live Forever in Paradise on Earth, c. 24: "Are We Under the Ten Commandments?" Author Farr, in his book *God*, Blood and Society, 73, sees this as a contradiction. In his view, by arguing that Christ's New Covenant abrogated the Mosaic law "(t)he clear implication is that the whole

law for a specific reason. It illustrates, for them, a continued determination on the part of God to view blood as sacred and to 'withhold it from human consumption.'[24] Described as a 'covenant concerning the sanctity of human life'[25] which came into force after Noah left the Ark, the holding of blood as sacred became a formal obligation imposed on the ancient nation of Israel and was further maintained during and after the arrival of Christ.

This prohibition on the consumption of blood was, according to Witnesses, intrinsic to the morality of first-century Jews. They point to the account of John 6: 53 where Jesus explained, in a figurative way,[26] to his disciples (who were Jews) that they needed to eat his flesh and drink his blood to be saved. Many found his speech to be 'shocking' (verse 60) and stopped following him.[27] The simple mention of drinking human blood, though common among the nations around them,[28] was sufficiently repulsive to immediately turn away from Christ those Jews who had begun accepting his teachings. The doctrine of transubstantiation (where it is believed that the bread and wine are literally transformed into the blood and flesh of Christ during Mass) was only adopted by the Roman Church in AD 1215.[29]

---

of the old law is abrogated, including the pre-Mosaic components," which would include the covenant with Noah. However, this seems to be incorrect for nowhere in their literature do the Witnesses take such a position. They view the covenant made with Noah as a covenant made with all of mankind, at a time when the nation of Israel did not exist. With the abrogation of the Mosaic law, the Noahic covenant remained untouched and continues to be valid; see Jehovah's Witnesses and the Question of Blood, *infra* note 43, 7.

[24] Davis, The Westminster Dictionary of the Bible, 77: "(…) the blood of animals was used in all offerings for sin, and the blood of beasts killed on the hunt or slaughtered for food was poured out and covered with earth, because withheld by God from man's consumption and reserved for the purposes of atonement."

[25] "One Reason for God's Vengeance," The Watchtower, 376.

[26] Jehovah's Witnesses understand this passage to have a symbolic meaning. See "Bread of Life" Available for All," The Watchtower, 18.

[27] Jehovah's Witnesses and the Question of Blood, *infra* note 43, 10.

[28] See *infra* notes 50, 51, 52, 53, 54 and accompanying text.

[29] The doctrine of transubstantiation was proclaimed in AD 1215 at the Lateran Council. Before that

While Witnesses believe that the Mosaic Law ceased to be in effect with the death of Christ, they nevertheless believe that Christians continue to be subjected to the prohibition on blood. The reason for this is that the prohibition on the consumption of blood was directly addressed by a council of apostles and elders of the early Christian church in Jerusalem a few years after the death of Christ. The issue brought before this council was whether Gentiles, who had converted to the Christian faith, were obliged to conform to the Mosaic Law. This issue caused a sharp debate among the members of the church of Antioch[30] and warranted sending the disciples Paul and Barnabas to submit the dispute to the council of apostles and elders in Jerusalem, for settlement. According to Acts 15:29, after hearing from the interested parties, the council arrived at the following decision: "It seemed good to the Holy Spirit and to us not to burden you with anything beyond the following requirements: You are to abstain from food sacrificed to idols, from blood, from the meat of strangled animals and from sexual immorality. You will do well to avoid these things."[31]

The Gentiles who had converted to Christianity were not to be subjected to the Mosaic Law, but only to the requirements mentioned above. This decision is often referred to as the "apostolic decree." Certain Bible commentators view it as stemming from the early prohibition on the consumption of blood given to Noah since the command given to Noah predated Moses. For example, John Wesley, (founder of Methodism, 1703-1791), referring to Acts 15:29, gave six reasons, including the prohibition given to Noah, why the consumption of blood "was never permitted the children of God from the beginning of the world."[32] Sir Isaac Newton, (physicist and mathematician, 1642-1727) in reference to the decision of

---

time, the words of Christ – "this is my body" (Luke 22:19) were understood to be figurative. See Binns, Innocent III, 172; Tannahill, Flesh & Blood, 77-84.

30 Acts 15:2: "This brought Paul and Barnabas into sharp dispute and debate with them."

31 Acts 15:28, 29.

32 Wesley, Explanatory Notes upon the New Testament.

the council of Jerusalem, viewed the prohibition "as being an earlier law of God, imposed not on the sons of Abraham only, but on all nations, while they lived together in Shinar under the dominion of Noah."[33] Bible commentator, Andrew Fuller, also held the view that the apostolic decree was to be viewed as a reinforcement of the prohibition given to Noah: "Here is also a special grant, which does not appear to have been given before: not only the herbs of the field, but the animals, are given to man for food. It is however accompanied with a special exception with regard to blood, which is the life. This, being forbidden to Noah, appears also to have been forbidden to all mankind; nor ought this prohibition to be treated as belonging to the ceremonies of the Jewish dispensation. It was not only enjoined before that dispensation existed, but was enforced upon the Gentile Christians by the decrees of the apostles, Acts xv. 20."[34]

Some Bible commentators did not agree. They believed that the "apostolic decree" found at Acts 15:29 was really "intended to obviate essential repugnance of legal Jews to Gentile customs."[35] However, the prevailing view of Bible commentators of the 18th and 19th century, with the exception of the Church of

---

33 Newton, The Chronology of Ancient Kingdoms Amended, 184: "This law was ancienter than the days of Moses being given to Noah and his sons, long before the days of Abraham: and therefore when the Apostles and Elders in the Council at Jerusalem declared that the Gentiles were not obliged to be circumcised and keep the law of Moses, they excepted this law of abstaining from blood, and things strangled, as being an earlier law of God, imposed not on the sons of Abraham only, but on all nations, while they lived together in Shinar under the dominion of Noah: and of the same kind is the law of abstaining from meats offered to idols or false Gods, and from fornication."

34 Fuller, Complete Works of the Rev. Andrew Fuller, With a Memoir Of His Life , *supra* note 22, 363.

35 Moeller, History of the Christian Church AD 1-600, 58; See also Milner, The History of the Church of Christ, 24, footnote: "to abstain from things strangled, and from blood, was necessary, in order to have any intercourse with Jews;" Calvin, Commentaries on The First Book of Moses called Genesis, 294: "For the apostles, in commanding the Gentiles to observe this rite, for a short time, did not intend to inject a scruple into their consciences;" Crosby (annotated by), The New Testament in Both Authorized and Revised Versions, 295: "So there were two reasons why the Gentiles Christians should abstain from these – that they might not be drawn into idolatry, and that they might not unnecessarily shock their brethren, the Jewish Christians."

Rome, was that this decree was to be binding on all Christians.[36] Those who advocate this position point to the Bible itself as it indicates that the decision of the council of Jerusalem was to be considered binding on all Christians. In fact, this decision was sent by letter to the congregation of Antioch[37] and eventually to the other congregations. Several years later, the disciple James, who had participated in this early decision, referred to the prohibition on blood as a binding provision for all "Gentile believers."[38] There is no evidence in the Bible indicating that this decision was ever rescinded.[39] The Latin Church, however, eventually abandoned the rule of abstaining "from blood and from things strangled" mainly due to the influence of St. Augustine (Bishop of Hippo, 354-430) who taught that this precept was given to Christians only while the Gentile Church was not yet settled.[40]

---

[36] See for example Schaff, A select Library of Nicene and Post-Nicene Fathers, 2:25. In his Lecture IV, S. Cyrill refers to the apostolic decree as "a Catholic epistle to all the Gentiles, that they should *abstain* first *from things offered to idols*, and then *from blood* also and *from things strangled*." [Emphasis added] The footnote to this comment states: "The prohibition of blood and things strangled has continued to the present day in the Eastern Church, though already disregarded by the Latins in the time of S. Augustine." McGarvey, A Commentary on Acts of Apostles: "There was room for no other conclusion than the one which James deduced, that they should impose on the Gentiles, so far as the class or restrictions under consideration were concerned, only those *necessary* things which were necessary independent of the Mosaic law. Idolatry, with all the pollutions connected with it, was known to be sinful before the law of Moses was given; and so was fornication. The eating of blood, and, by implication, of strangled animals, whose blood was still in them, was forbidden to the whole world in the family of Noah. In the restrictions here proposed by James, therefore, there is not the slightest extension of the law of Moses, but a mere enforcement upon the Gentiles of rules of conduct which have ever been binding, and were to be perpetual. They are binding to-day as they were then. To deny this would be to despise the combined authority of all the apostles, when enjoining upon the Gentile world, of which we form a part, restrictions which they pronounce *necessary*." [Emphasis added] See also De Courcelles, "Diatriba de Esu Sanguinis Inter Christianos," 971; Benson, The Holy Bible, Containing the Old and new Testaments, 43.

[37] Acts 15:30, 31: "The men were sent off and went down to Antioch, where they gathered the church together and delivered the letter. The people read it and were glad for its encouraging message."

[38] Acts 21:25: "As for the Gentile believers, we have written to them our decision that they should abstain from food sacrificed to idols, from blood, from the meat of strangled animals and from sexual immorality."

[39] Pirie, A Dissertation on Baptism and Letters on the Sinai Covenant 241-79; Clarke, The New Testament of our Lord and Savior Jesus Christ, 806-12.

[40] Schaff, A Select Library of Nicene and Post-Nicene Fathers, *supra* note 36, 14:395. See also *infra* note 56.

Jehovah Witnesses have adhered to the "apostolic decree" from their early beginnings. In 1892, *Zion's Watch Tower*, the predecessor to their periodical *The Watch Tower*, commented on the decision handed down by the council of Jerusalem consisting of the apostles and elders of the early Christian Church.[41] Since that time, Jehovah's Witnesses have consistently held the view that the prohibition by God on the eating of blood has been in force from the time of Noah and continues to be valid and binding to this day. For them, it is a matter of obedience to God and respect for his role as Creator. They reason: "Blood has a special meaning. It stands for life provided by the Creator. By treating blood as special, the people showed dependence on him for life."[42]

Early Christians refused to consume blood

Witnesses point to the fact that early Christians adhered closely to the apostolic decree of Acts 15:29, even when their life was at stake.[43] This is confirmed by historical records which indicate that early Christians at times faced hardships because of their uncompromisable belief that they could not consume blood under any circumstances. Though they lived in a society which consumed both animal and human blood for either medical or religious reasons or as part of their diet, early Christians conscientiously refused to participate in any activity which entailed the consumption of blood.

Even under pressure, the record shows that early Christians refused to violate the "apostolic decree" of Acts 15:29. For example, when persecuted, Christians would sometimes be starved and be then given food containing blood. Tertullian (Christian apologist, approx. AD 160-230) describes these ordeals as

---

41 "The Apostolic Council," Zion's Watch Tower, 350.

42 How Can Blood Save Your Life?, *supra* note 5, 6.

43 Jehovah's Witnesses and the Question of Blood, 13-14; "Early Christians Under Roman Rule," The Watchtower, 137.

follows: "At the trials of Christians you offer them sausages filled with blood. You are convinced, of course, that the very thing which you try to make them deviate from the right way is unlawful for them."[44]

Commenting on the writings of Tertullian, John Dalderby (Bishop of Lincoln, 1300-1320) concluded that "the Primitive Christians scrupulously complied with the decree pronounced by the Apostles at Jerusalem, in abstaining from things strangled and from blood."[45]

The importance early Christians attached to the apostolic decree is also seen in their response to false accusations.[46] Faced with the outrageous accusation that Christians ate their own children, Minucius Felix (Christian apologist, 2nd century) responded, in his *Octavius*, that such a charge was impossible since, for Christians, "it is not lawful either to see or to hear of homicide; and so much do we shrink from human blood, that we do not use the blood even of eatable animals in our food."[47]

Tertullian, for his part, responded to this accusation by reminding his accusers of their own practice of wanting to eat the "(s)tag (which) has rolled in the blood of a gladiator. The very bellies of the bears, still stuffed with undigested human flesh, are the object of their search." He pointed out, as did Minucius Felix, that Christians did not even eat animal flesh that had not been properly bled, much less would they eat human flesh. He stated: "Let your unnatural ways blush before the Christians. We do not even have the blood of animals at our meals, for these consist of ordinary food. This is why we refrain from eating the

---

44 *Ibid.*

45 Dalderby, The Ecclesiastical History of the Second and Third Centuries, 146.

46 Regarding false accusations against early Christians see Arnold, The Early Christians After the Death of the Apostles, 89-90 regarding the accusation of eating their own children.

47 Roberts, The Ante-Nicene Fathers. Translations of The Writings of the Fathers down to AD 325, *infra* note 52, 192.

meat of any animals which have been strangled or that die of themselves, lest we be in any way contaminated with blood, even if it is hidden in the flesh."[48]

The defense given by Tertullian against the charge of cannibalism was also used by other Christians. For example, Eusebius (Christian theologian, approx. 260-340), in his *Ecclesiastical History*, speaks of a martyr named Biblias who, before being tortured to death, refuted the false accusation of infanticide and cannibalism by saying: "(H)ow could such as these devour children, who considered it unlawful even to taste the blood of irrational animals?"[49]

The Christian position on the consumption of blood stood out in sharp contrast with the usages of blood as practiced at that time. In fact, the use of blood was common in all walks of life during this period. Tertullian speaks of the Scythians in whose case, "blood was taken from the arms and tasted by both parties in forming a treaty," or how it was the custom of certain of their tribes "for every deceased member to be eaten by his relatives."[50] Roman historian Sallust (86-34 BC) tells of conspirators being bound by a covenant of blood.[51] Minucius Felix speaks to those who would "devour the wild beasts from the arena, besmeared and stained with blood, or fattened with the limbs or the entrails of men."[52] Blood was also sometimes prescribed as a cure for epilepsy.[53] This would explain Tertullian's comments about those who "with greedy thirst, at a show in the arena, take the fresh blood of wicked criminals as it runs down from their throats and carry it off to heal their epilepsy."[54]

---

[48] Arbesmann (transl.), Tertullian Apologetical Works and Minucius Felix Octavius., *infra* note 50, 32-3.

[49] Eusebius, An Ecclesiastical History, 200; See also Hall, "Women Among the Early Martyrs," 11.

[50] Arbesmann, Tertullian Apologetical Works and Minucius Felix Octavius, *supra* note 48, 32.

[51] *Ibid.*, 386, footnote 7.

[52] Roberts, The Ante-Nicene Fathers. Translations of The Writings of the Fathers down to AD 325, 192.

[53] Arbesmann, Tertullian Apologetical Works and Minucius Felix Octavius, *supra* note 48, 386, footnote 9.

[54] *Ibid.*, 32.

It is uncertain until when the early Christians maintained this firm stand regarding the consumption of blood.[55] However, early records reveal that by the time of St. Augustine some Christians in Africa were not observing the prohibition as the eating of unbled animals was common place amongst them.[56] Augustine himself was of the view that the apostolic decree was of a temporary nature and would not be binding on all future Christians.[57] With time, the Latin Church followed his opinion.[58] The Eastern Church, though, maintained observance of the "apostolic decree" as can be seen in Canon LXVII of the Council in Trullo, known as the Quinisext Council (AD 692): "The divine Scripture commands us to abstain from blood, from things strangled, and from fornication. Those therefore who on account of a dainty stomach prepare by any art for food the blood of any animal, and so eat it, we punish suitably. If any one henceforth venture to eat in any way the blood of an animal, if he be a clergyman, let him be deposed; if a layman, let him be cut off."[59]

---

[55] "We further see that, at the time of the Synod of Gangra, the rule of the Apostolic Synod with regard to blood and things strangled was still in force." This comment was made regarding the second Canon set forth at the Synod of Gangra (AD 325-381) which states: "If any one shall condemn him who eats flesh, which is without blood and has not been offered to idols nor strangled, and is faithful and devout, as though the man were without hope [of salvation] because of his eating, let him be anathema." Percival, The seven Ecumenical Councils of the Undivided Church, 14:92.

[56] Dods, The Works of Aurelius Augustine, Bishop of Hippo, 5:541: In his *Contra Faustum*, Augustine states that: "no Christian feels bound to abstain from thrushes or small birds because their blood has not been poured out, or from hares because they are killed by a stroke on the neck without shedding their blood. Any who still are afraid to touch these things are laughed at by the rest: so general is the conviction of the truth, that 'not what entereth into the mouth defileth you, but what cometh out of it'; that evil lies in the commission of sin, and not in the nature of any food in ordinary use."

[57] In Augustin's reply to Faustus the Manichaean, he argues that the apostolic decree was given to Christians only while the Church was not yet settled, see *Ibid.*, 540. See also comments by Percival, The Seven Ecumenical Councils of the Undivided Church, *supra* note 55, 395, notes on Canon LXVII.

[58] The apostolic decree all but lost its meaning for the Latin Church even though there is evidence that as late as the eighth century, Pope Gregory III (AD 731) "forbade the eating of blood or things strangled under threat of a penance of forty days." See Percival, The seven Ecumenical Councils of the Undivided Church, *supra* note 55, 93, notes on Canon II. See also Robinson, The Life of Otto Apostle of Pomerania, 87 where Otto Apostle of Pomerania (1060-1139) preached that Christians should not eat the blood of animals.

[59] Percival, The seven Ecumenical Councils of the Undivided Church, *supra* note 55, 395. See also *supra* note 36 and accompanying text.

In the western world the advent of the Reformation produced many Bible commentators and scholars who began advocating obedience to the apostolic decree found in Acts 15:28. Martin Luther (1483-1546) for example, led the way when he commented on this decree by saying: "Now if we want to have a church that conforms to this council … we must teach and insist that henceforth no prince, lord, burgher, or peasant eat geese, doe, stag, or pork cooked in blood… And burghers and peasants must abstain especially from red sausage and blood sausage."[60]

Other Bible commentators followed suit. Some produced lengthy treatises on this issue in order to refute what they considered "weak and ungrounded, very unlearned reasons, for believing" the "apostolic decree" to have been repealed.[61] Alexander Pirie's early 19th century dissertation addressed in detail the many arguments advanced by those who advocated eating blood. Using Bible references and logic, he argued in favor of observing the "apostolic decree."[62] Adam Clarke, in his Bible commentary of Acts 15:28, included Dr Delaney's article which presented forceful arguments as to why the apostolic decree was still binding on Christians.[63]

Interestingly, in his commentary on Genesis, Clarke invoked scientific and medical research to support the prohibition on the consumption of blood. Both Genesis[64] and Leviticus[65] taught that blood was prohibited because 'life was in the

---

[60] Gritsch, Luther's Works, 28.

[61] Clarke, The New Testament of our Lord and Savior Jesus Christ, *supra* note 39, 812.

[62] Pirie, A Dissertation on Baptism and Letters on the Sinai Covenant; Together With an Inquiry Into the Lawfulness of Eating Blood, *supra* note 39, 241-79. In his dissertation, Pirie justifies his long discussion of the question by the fact that "disputes on this point have run high, and many arguments have been offered on both sides of the question."

[63] Clarke, The New Testament of our Lord and Savior Jesus Christ, *supra* note 39, 806-12. For a more recent comment see also The Interpreter's Bible, 549-50.

[64] Genesis 9:4: "But you must not eat meat that has its lifeblood still in it."

[65] Leviticus 17:11: "For the life of a creature is in the blood (…)."

blood' and this life belonged to God. Referring to Harvey's experiments in 1628 on the circulation of blood and research done by Hunter, professor of anatomy, regarding the 'vitality' of blood, Clarke argued that scientific research supported the view that blood "possesses a *living principle*, and that life of the whole body is derived from it."[66]

Some physicians viewed the new practice of transfusing blood as contrary to the "apostolic decree." Bartolomeo Santinelle, a 17th century Italian physician, wrote: "Although indeed the prohibition of the use of blood would have in view only that man should not eat it, for which reason it would seem to pertain less to our cause, nonetheless the purpose of that injunction is contrary to today's transfusion [practice], so that the one who employs it would appear to oppose God who extends clemency."[67]

Thomas Bartholin (1616-1680), anatomist and mathematician considered those using human blood to be 'sinning gravely.' He wrote: "Similar is the receiving of alien blood from a cut vein, either through the mouth, a thing that is recommended for senile hectic fever, or by instruments of transfusion, a thing that, contrived through the devising of the moderns, already has come almost into disuse, when it scarcely has become known in the world. The authors of this operation are held in terror by the divine law, by which eating of blood is prohibited."[68]

Jehovah's Witnesses teach and assist their members

The theological reasons explained above regarding the prohibition on the consumption of blood form the basis of Witnesses' refusal of blood transfusion therapy. From their early beginnings Jehovah's Witnesses considered themselves

---

[66] Clark, The Holy Bible, Containing the Old and New Testaments, *supra* note 11, 565.

[67] Santinelli, Confusio Transfusionis, sive Confutatio Operationis Transfundentis Sanguinem de Individuo ad Individuum (A Confounding of Transfusion, or A Refutation of the Operation of Transfusing Blood from Individual to Individual), 130-1.

to be under divine commandment to abstain from blood, whether as food or otherwise, and so educated their members through the magazine *The Watchtower*, as well as through other publications. In 1892, they discussed the apostolic decree found at Acts 15:28, 29 regarding the necessity to "abstain from blood, from the meat of strangled animals," and considered it to be a repetition of an earlier law of God: "The same command was given to Noah."[69] In their view, this law spanned the period of time from the new beginning of mankind after the flood, right up to and beyond the establishment of the Christian Church.

Subsequently, in a 1909 article discussing the apostolic decree, the Witnesses reasoned that "there may be other, sanitary, reasons connected with the matter, which are not yet known to us."[70] They believed that God's law on this matter, even if not completely understood at that time, was for the eventual benefit of mankind.[71] In the same article, the fact that blood "was made a symbol of life" under the Law of Moses, and could only be used on the altar for the atonement of sins, was highlighted. It was forbidden to consume it. For Witnesses, it was not difficult to observe this prohibition since, "nearly all the butchering for our markets is in harmony with the Jewish regulations."[72]

In 1927, they again considered the subject by describing the command given to Noah regarding blood as a "covenant … made with Noah and applied to him

---

[68] Bartholin, De Sanguinis Abusu Disputatio (A Disputation Concerning the Misuse of Blood), 140-3.

[69] "The Apostolic Council," Zion's Watch Tower, *supra* note 41, 350.

[70] "Settling Doctrinal Differences," Zion's Watch Tower, 117.

[71] They eventually took the view that the 'other reasons connected with the matter' related to the "practice of blood transfusion." See "By Man's Way or by God's Way – Which?," The Watchtower, 721, where, regarding the 'reasons connected with the matter' mentioned in the 1909 reference, it is stated: "Today, fifty-eight years since then, those reasons are becoming more and more known because of medical experiences with the widespread use of transfusions. Now, what would you think of a modern medical practice that, in one year, directly kills 16,000 in a land, and leaves still more thousands infected with deadly diseases, while at the same time other thousands survive the process? That is the case with the practice of blood transfusion."

[72] "Settling Doctrinal Differences," Zion's Watch Tower, *supra* note 70, 117.

and every living creature."[73] Since blood transfusion therapy had not yet become a standard medical practice, it would be several years before the issue regarding blood came up again in their literature.

Near the end of World War II, when blood transfusion was developing into a standard medical practice,[74] the Witnesses took a definite stand on the issue of whether or not this therapy violated God's law. Before the end of the War, on July 1st, 1945, a lengthy article, in their periodical *The Watchtower*, addressed the issue of the sanctity of blood with regard to blood transfusions.[75] The article reiterated what had been previously stated in the December 1927 issue of the same magazine, that the covenant "regarding life," which included the prohibition on eating blood made with Noah, was an "everlasting covenant" which continued to apply to all humans.[76] They argued that even though the Mosaic covenant, incorporating the same prohibition, had been abolished with the coming of Christ, the covenant with Noah continued to be valid.[77] Referring to the "apostolic decree" of Acts 15:28, 29 the article stated: "They wrote such instruction concerning blood and carcasses not drained of blood, not because Christians were under the Mosaic law covenant, but because they were under the covenant made after the flood with Noah and which embraced all mankind."[78]

Relying in part on an excerpt from *The Encyclopedia Americana* that traced the history of transfusion from its early beginnings, the article concluded that the prohibition on the consumption of blood also applied to blood transfusions.[79]

---

[73] "One Reason for God's Vengeance," The Watchtower, *supra* note 25.

[74] Spence, "Transfusion and Surgery," 1105.

[75] "Immovable for the Right Worship," The Watchtower, 195.

[76] "One Reason for God's Vengeance," The Watchtower, *supra* note 25.

[77] See Romans 7:6; Galatians 3:23-25.

[78] "Immovable for the Right Worship," The Watchtower, *supra* note 75, 199.

[79] *Ibid.*, 200. The excerpt is taken from the 1929 revised edition of The Encyclopedia Americana, vol. 4 and states: "Transfusion of blood dates as far back as the time of the ancient Egyptians. The earliest reported case is that practiced on Pope Innocent VIII in 1492. The operation cost the lives of three youths and the Pontiff's life was not saved. Great strides in the research and practice of transfusion on

Witnesses adopted the view that whether it be eating blood or having it transfused directly into the body, abstaining from all such practices was a "vital matter" for those who seek God's approval.[80] To manifest their firm decision to refuse blood therapy, as early as 1950 some Witnesses began to carry a card in their wallet requesting "No blood transfusion."[81] It has now become a practice for all Witnesses to carry on their person an *Advance Medical Directive* that directs that no allogeneic blood or blood products be administered under any circumstances.[82]

This religious stand brought them into conflict with the medical community at a time when paternalism was the norm and patient autonomy was often given little consideration. The view held by Jehovah's Witnesses was seen by many as unreasonable and even suicidal. However, the Witnesses, ever convinced that this prohibition comes from God and could only be for the good of humankind, constantly sought evidence of possible dangers associated with blood transfusion therapy. Whenever information on the hazards of blood transfusion became

---

animals were made after Harvey's discovery of the circulation of the blood in the middle of the 17th century. Physicians in Germany, England and France were especially active in the work of blood transfusion after this discovery. They reasoned that as the blood is the principal medium by which the body is nourished, transfusion, therefore, is a quicker and shorter road to feed an ill-nourished body than eating food which turns to blood after several changes. So transfusion was thought of not only as a cure, but also as a rejuvenator. Attempts were then made to cure various diseases, such as fevers, leprosy, insanity and hydrophobia. Lamb's blood was used for transfusions into human beings with varying success. Curious to relate, the Faculty of Medicine of Paris refused to recognize Harvey's discovery and also opposed any progress made in the art of transfusion. They persecuted those who were active in the research work of transfusion. It was in the end of the 18th and in the beginning of the 19th century that the most active work in establishing transfusion as a surgical procedure after hemorrhage was done." See also "Is Blood Transfusion Scriptural?," Awake!, 25. In their more recent publication How Can Blood Save Your Life? *supra* note 5, 6.

80 "Immovable for the Right Worship," The Watchtower, *supra* note 75, 201.

81 "An "Exclusion Clause" Recommended," The Watchtower, 524. The article relates the experience of a nurse in a large hospital who was one of Jehovah's Witnesses and who had observed first hand transfusion practices. She wrote: "Be it known that it is becoming more prevalent to give blood transfusion during quite simple operations, and the only knowledge the patient may have of it is when asked to have friends and relatives replace it in the blood bank. To avoid this an exclusion clause should be inserted in the hospital release contract before signing for operation. I carry an identification card in my wallet marked "No blood transfusion" in red ink and bearing my signature."

82 See page 144 for current Advance Medical Directive carried by baptized members of the Jehovah's Witness faith.

available, they published it in their literature. As early as 1948 they pointed to findings by Dr Richard B. Capps that over 20% of patients receiving blood were being contaminated with the hepatitis virus. This research also alerted the public to the danger that such a virus could present in pooled blood.[83]

Witnesses also circulated published comments of the few doctors who opposed the practice of blood transfusion. For example, in a 1949 article, Dr Alonzo J. Shadman claimed to have practiced medicine for 40 years without ever transfusing blood, and yet he "never had a patient any the worse for not having received it." He compared the relatively new practice of blood transfusion to the old practice of bloodletting, known as phlebotomy. He realized that his opinion was dissident and unpopular since, at that time, the practice was accepted "by physicians and laity as the 'thing to do' and who had the temerity to question orthodox medicine in the great and enlightened year of 1948."[84]

During the following decades, blood transfusion therapy became firmly entrenched as a standard practice in the medical community. As a result, Jehovah's Witnesses' objection to this therapy increasingly became an object of controversy.[85] In their defense, they published a voluminous amount of related material that received worldwide circulation. This information, intended for the benefit of their members as well as the public, addressed the theological, ethical, legal and medical aspects of the decision to opt for alternative treatment to blood transfusion therapy. In 1961 they published a 64-page booklet entitled *Blood,*

---

[83] "Dangers of Blood Transfusion," Awake!, 12.

[84] "Blood Transfusion – One Doctor's Opinion," Awake!, 12. Other doctors did, with time, report on the dangers of blood transfusions. See, for example, Unger "Medical-Legal Aspects of Blood Transfusion," 237, which states: "The mortality from blood transfusion equals that from either anesthesia or appendectomy. In the London area there has been reported one death for every 13,000 bottles of blood transfused."

[85] An early article discussion their objection to blood transfusion is found in Ford, "The Refusal of Blood Transfusions by Jehovah's Witnesses," 3.

Medicine and the Law of God. Subsequent updates in 1977,[86] and again in 1990,[87] with the latest medical research were again widely distributed.

Between 1950 and 1997 they published over 130 articles in their magazine *The Watchtower* and at least 300 articles in the magazine *Awake!,* all relating to the question of blood transfusion. Many of these articles presented up-to-date scientific research on the dangers of blood transfusions as well as possible alternatives.[88] In all these articles, they consistently maintained their objection to the use of blood transfusion under any circumstances. Several accounts were published of individuals who had succeeded in convincing doctors to respect their conscientious objection to blood transfusion therapy, and the results.[89] During the same time, they also vigorously fought legal battles in various countries to establish the right for patients to make autonomous medical decisions.[90] One of their most remarkable accomplishments was the establishment of a network of Hospital Liaison Committees in major centers around the world whose main task

---

86 Jehovah's Witnesses and the Question of Blood, *supra* note 43. A special campaign by Jehovah's Witnesses to distribute this edition to 370,000 U.S. physicians and hospital officials, one million registered nurses, 320,000 lawyers and judges, as well as to professionals in countries such as Canada, England, Finland, France, Germany, Italy, Japan, Sweden is reported in "Blood Transfusions: Why Many Are Taking a Fresh Look," Awake!, 16.

87 How Can Blood Save Your Life?, *supra* note 5.

88 Between 1950 and 1997, over 90 articles were printed regarding the dangers of blood transfusion therapy and over 40 articles were printed regarding alternative treatment. These articles received wide circulation since the Awake! circulation grew from 3,000,000 (in 21 languages) in 1960 to over 18,000,000 (in 81 languages) in 1997. Circulation of The Watchtower grew from more than 3,000,000 (in 58 languages) in 1960 to over 20,900,000 (in 125 languages) in 1997. (Circulation of these magazines appears in every issue.)

89 Between 1950 and 1997, over 80 articles were printed regarding cases where individuals recovered after refusing blood transfusions and asking for alternative treatment.

90 W. Glen How, General Counsel for Jehovah's Witnesses, fought many legal battles in Canada, the United States and other countries, defending Witness patients when doctors and hospitals petitioned Courts to force blood transfusion therapy on them. In 1960, in the Canadian Bar Journal, he published a scathing attack on the practice of blood transfusion describing it as a practice "founded more on mysticism and showmanship than on scientific proof and really curative value" and predicting that, because of the dangers involved, it would go "the way of bloodletting into the limbo of desuetude." How, "Religion Medicine and Law," 365-432.

is to assist fellow Witnesses finding themselves in a hospital setting due to sickness or injury. These committees worked to develop a local and international network of medical specialists willing to treat Witness patients using medical alternatives to blood transfusions. This meant supplying doctors with medical, ethical, legal and theological information to help them understand the objection of Jehovah's Witnesses to blood transfusion, and assisting them in offering treatment which does not violate the beliefs of these patients.

2. Overview of the Use of Blood in Medicine

We were governed by the best light we had; we thought we were right, and so we are justified. –

J.W. Estes[91]

The analysis of the objection by an individual to a particular form of medical treatment requires understanding the nature of, and the reason for, the objection, as well as the medical treatment itself. In the case of blood transfusion, this is particularly important in view of the miraculous, indeed almost mystic life saving properties assigned to blood from the earliest times of antiquity. It involves looking not only at the history of blood transfusion, but also at earlier medical practices using blood.

Early use of blood in medicine

Early medical writings indicate a widespread use of blood in the practice of medicine. Pliny The Elder (AD 23-79), author of the celebrated *Natural History*,[92] refers to the Pharaohs of Egypt who, when stricken with leprosy, bathed in human blood as a remedy. He describes epileptics who found it "efficient" to drink the warm blood gushing from the open wounds of gladiators, in effect drinking 'their living soul.' He enumerates several ailments that could be treated by administering the blood of specific animals in a variety of ways.

---

[91] Estes, "George Washington and the Doctors: Treating America's First Superhero," 43-57.

[92] Considered to be the first encyclopedia, Natural History was completed in AD 77 and dedicated to Titus. It was divided into 37 books and was an attempt to gather older scattered material on a variety of topics including medicine. A novel feature of this work was that Pliny named authors and titles of books he relied upon. Though it contained both factual and fictional data, including unsupported claims, fables, and exaggerations, Natural History was an authority on scientific matters up to the Middle Ages and helped shape scientific and medical theory during that time. For a detailed history of bloodletting, see Garrison, "The History of Bloodletting," 432-7, 498-501.

Pliny also refers to the age-old practice of phlebotomy, or bloodletting, the origin of which is unknown, but is believed to have been practiced by the Egyptians from as early as 2500 BC[93] Primitive cultures are believed to have used sharpened flints, the teeth of fish, as well as thorns to let blood.[94] The practice became a "sort of therapeutic sheet-anchor" in medicine for millenniums.[95] Greek physician Hippocrates (460-377 BC), considered by many as the father of medicine, referred to bloodletting within the context of humoral medicine, which taught that all sicknesses resulted from an imbalance of the fluids of the body.[96] Through the conquests of Alexander the Great, medical knowledge regarding bloodletting, as well as the practice itself, spread to both the Persian and Hindu worlds.[97] Aulus Cornelius Celsus (first century Roman encyclopedist) wrote "to let blood by incising a vein is no novelty, what is novel is that there should be scarcely any malady in which blood may not be let."[98] Druidical medicine in Britain included bloodletting which was "regulated by the moon's age."[99] In Papua New Guinea, healers treated headaches by shooting six-inch arrows from small bows into the head as a form of bloodletting.[100]

Greek physician, Galen of Pergamun (AD 129-216), expanded on the

---

[93] L'Ancien, Histoire Naturelle, Books 26 and 28. That Egyptians may have practiced bleeding is seen from an illustration on a tomb near ancient Memphis which shows some being bled from the neck and from the foot. See Garrison, "The History of Bloodletting," *supra* note 92, 432.

[94] Garrison, An Introduction to the History of Medicine, 28. See also Ortiz de Montellano, Aztec Medicine, Health, and Nutrition, 149, 179.

[95] Garrison, An Introduction to the History of Medicine, *supra* note 94, 29.

[96] According to the Hippocratic Corpus health was equilibrium and illness an upset. Bodily fluids or 'humors' (Bile, phlegm, blood and black bile) were being kept in balance. For discussion see Porter, The greatest Benefit to Mankind, 56-8.

[97] For bloodletting among the Arabs (known as cupping) see Islamic Medical Wisdom the Tibb Al-A'Imma, trans. Batool Ispahany, 64-143. For bloodletting among the Hindus, see History of Medicine in India from Antiquity to AD 1000, 329.

[98] Celsus de Medicina, 1:155.

[99] Garrison, An Introduction to the History of Medicine, *supra* note 94, 169.

[100] Burton-Bradley, A History of Medicine in Papua New Guinea, 5.

concept of humoral medicine by stating that human health required an equilibrium between the four main bodily fluids, or humours: blood, yellow bile, black bile, and phlegm. To reestablish this equilibrium, he resorted to bloodletting which played an important part in his practice.[101] While much of Galen's medical knowledge, though very influential, proved to be inaccurate, he did, however, correctly determine that arteries (from the Greek *aer*-air and *terein*-to conserve) were filled with blood and not with air from the lungs, as was previously believed.

This was a time when doctors did not understand the true nature of disease. The existence of germs, bacteria and viruses was unknown. In place of scientific research, ignorance and superstition played a dominant role in the continuing practice of bloodletting. Bloodletting became the longest enduring inefficient and often dangerous medical therapy ever developed. The physician was guided by his own personal experience at the bedside of a patient or by the experience of his predecessors, thus perpetrating useless and dangerous remedies. The treatment was administered, and if the patient didn't die, it was deemed to be successful. Nevertheless, bloodletting managed to survive antiquity and actually flourished to become the standard and most popular medical therapy during the middle ages.

"There is no remedy in the world capable of such miracles as bloodletting," boasted Guy Patin (1601-1672), French physician and staunch supporter of bloodletting, as he proceeded to make a seventh incision in a vein of his own arm to cure a cold.[102] Bloodletting was prescribed for every imaginable illness and disorder, even including hemorrhages. It was relied upon as the "queen of remedies."[103] Its use went even beyond the boundaries of medicine and was

---

[101] "Galen of Pergamum" Encyclopoedia Britannica Online, http://members.eb.com/bol/topic?eu=36532&sctn=1.

[102] "Il n'y a pas de remède au monde qui fassent tant de miracles que la saignée." Héritier, La sève de l'homme, 19. The procedure for bloodletting involved tying a bandage around the arm to make the forearm veins swell up. The exposed vein was then opened with a lancet. This was called 'breathing a vein'. For a detailed description of the methods and instruments used see 167-72.

[103] Brockliss, The Medical World of Early Modern France , 159.

sometimes even administered as a form of punishment.[104] It was even administered to those who were not sick as a "preventive measure."[105] Those who dared oppose phlebotomy as a cure-all were described by Patin as 'wicked,' 'insane,' 'ignorant,' 'charlatans,' 'atheists,' and 'imposters.'[106] Certain astrological conditions were preferred for bloodletting, and calendars were even printed for that specific purpose.[107] Records indicate the practice to have been a lucrative one.[108] Guilds for surgeons and barber-surgeons were organized in France and England during the 13th and 14th centuries.[109] Bleeding was held in such high respect by British physicians that they named their pre-eminent journal

---

104 Pichon, Le Ménagier de Paris, 1:164. This is an account of a Parisian house wife who displeased her husband on three occasions and was punished with a bleed: "Dame, vous m'avez fait trois grands déplaisirs et courroux, si je peux vous ne m'en ferez pas un quatrième; et je sais bien que cela vous a fait faire du mauvais sang; il faut vous saigner. Il appelle le barbier et fait faire le feu. La dame lui dit :

-Sire, que voulez-vous faire? Je n'ai jamais été saignée.

-Tant pis, fait le seigneur, il vous faut commencer : les trois mauvaises actions que vous avez commises contre moi vous ont fait faire du mauvais sang.

Alors il lui fait chauffer le bras droit au feu, et quand il fut échauffé, il la fit saigner; elle saigna tant que le sang épais et vermeil sortit. Alors le seigneur la fit panser, et puis lui fait retirer l'autre bras hors de la robe. La dame commence à crier grâce. Mais ça ne l'avance à rien, car il la fit chauffer et saigner de ce second bras; et elle commença à saigner : il la tint ainsi si longtemps qu'elle s'évanouit et perdit la parole, et devint tout entière d'une pâleur mortelle."

105 "par précaution." Pichon, Le Ménagier de Paris, *supra* note 104, 42. Such blind faith and certitude of the usefulness of their therapy often caused physicians to be the object of public scorn. See for example Molière's play Le malade imaginaire and Dickens' Mudfog Papers.

106 Packard, "Guy Patin and the Medical profession in Paris in The Seventeenth Century," 358, 363-4. About Guy de la Brosse (physician to Louis XIII) who would rather die than be bled, Patin wrote in 1641: "The devil will bleed him in the other world, as merits a rascal, an atheist, an impostor, a homicide, and a public executioner such as he was."

107 Porter, The Greatest Benefit to Mankind, *supra* note 96, 115-6. Astrology was part of mainstream medicine, a practice going as far back as Hippocrates. It was believed that the motion of the planets has an influence on the human body and its diseases. Through the Middle Ages, princely courts often housed a physician-astrologer.

108 Héritier, La sève de l'homme, *supra* note 102, 26-9.

109 Garrison, An Introduction to the History of Medicine, *supra* note 94, 172. During this time period, surgeons formed a separate class from the physicians who looked down upon them. The surgeons were divided into two groups – the surgeon and the surgeon-barber. The surgeon was usually a cleric (known as the surgeon of the long robe) while the surgeon-barber was a lay barber (known as the surgeon of the short robe) and who had originally been trained for the purpose of bleeding and shaving the monks.

after the preferred surgical instrument used in phlebotomy: *The Lancet.*[110] The journal still carries the name.

While bloodletting continued to be in vogue on the Continent, often with the use of leaches (French doctors imported 41.5 million leaches in 1833 alone),[111] colonization brought the practice to America. The leading American advocate of bleeding was no doubt Benjamin Rush (1745-1813), physician and signee to the Declaration of Independence, known as the 'Prince of Bleeders.'[112] Believing that the human body contained 12,500-14,500 cc. of blood,[113] he promoted the use of the lancet in almost every case and even in cases where it had never before been used.[114] During the yellow-fever plague in Philadelphia in 1793, the worst in American history, casualties were so numerous that the city, then the nation's capital, was emptied and its government collapsed. Rush stayed behind to care for the sick and dying. His treatment included a massive dose of mercury and jalap, to produce diarrhea, which was then followed up with copious bleeding.[115] He would visit as many as a hundred patients in a day and the bleeding was so profuse that the blood, "from want of a sufficient number of bowls, was often

---

[110] The lancet was used for bloodletting by venesection. Other methods were arteriotomy, scarification with wet cupping and the use of leeches. For a detailed description and explanation of bloodletting methods see Seigworth, "Bloodletting Over the Centuries," 2024-7.

[111] Garrison, An Introduction to the History of Medicine, *supra* note 94, 409.

[112] Schmidt, "Transfusion In America In the Eighteenth And Nineteenth Centuries," 1319. See also Siddall, "Bloodletting in American Obstetric Practice, 1800-1945," 102. This article explains that bloodletting was also prevalent in obstetrics during the nineteenth century. Patients were bled for almost all of their "minor antenatal complaints, such as headaches, vertigo, nausea and vomiting, insomnia, apprehension, palpitation, muscle cramps, diarrhea, hemorrhoids, varicose veins, and swelling of the lower extremities." (105) Pregnant patients were even bled for hemorrhage. "The paradoxical treatment of hemorrhage in pregnancy by bloodletting was based on the logic that in producing a faint by venesection, the force of the patient's circulation was so reduced that clotting could take place, which in turn checked the hemorrhage." (106) To control a convulsive disorder called eclampsia a venesection of 900-1800 cc. was recommended in addition to shaving the patient's head so leeches could be applied to the scalp." (109)

[113] Siddall, "Bloodletting in American Obstetric Practice, 1800-1945," *supra* note 112, 102.

[114] Pepper, "Benjamin Rush," 599.

[115] Starr, Blood, An Epic History of Medicine and Commerce, 24.

allowed to flow upon the ground."[116] Convinced that his patients were surviving due to his treatment, he wrote his wife on September 13, 1793: "Yesterday was a day of triumph to mercury, jalap and bleeding. I am satisfied that they saved, in my hand only, nearly one hundred lives."[117] He would, however, have been of greater help to his patients if he had left them alone. It is known today that this plague was caused by the *Aëdes (Stegomyia) œgypti* mosquito, whose bite spreads yellow fever through a virus that follows its course and then leaves the body. Copious bleeding in these cases only weakened the body and hastened death.[118]

Benjamin Rush came under heavy criticism from a young journalist named William Cobbett who accused him of "puffing his treatment and failing to report deaths."[119] Rush successfully sued Cobbett. Following his conviction, Cobbett wrote: "On the 14th of December, on the same day, and in the very *same hour*, that a ruinous fine was imposed on me for endeavoring to put a stop to the practice of Rush, *General Washington was expiring under the operation of that very practice.*"[120] In effect, Washington, suffering from what appeared to be strep, was bled copiously and subsequently died. Bloodletting came under heavy criticism; some even suggesting that bloodletting be made a criminal offense. With time, the magic began to slowly fade.[121]

Surprisingly, bloodletting was still being recommended as a treatment in the United States in the early 1920s.[122] However, the discovery that microbes, not

---

116 Pepper, "Benjamin Rush," *supra* note 114, 599.

117 Butterfield, Letters of Benjamin Rush, 1793-1813, 2:663 quoted in Starr, Blood, An Epic History of Medicine and Commerce, *supra* note 115, 25.

118 Walter Reed (1851-1902) proved, through experimentation, that yellow fever was caused by the *Stegomyia* mosquito. See Garrison, An Introduction to the History of Medicine, *supra* note 94, 718-9.

119 Starr, Blood, An Epic History of Medicine and Commerce, *supra* note 115, 27.

120 *Ibid.*

121 Bryan, Jr, "Blood-Letting in American Medicine, 1830-1892," 516-9.

122 Osler, The Principles and Practice of Medicine, 102: "We employed it much more than we did a few years ago, but more often late in the disease than early. To bleed at the very onset in robust, healthy individuals in who disease sets in with great intensity and high fever is good practice."

humors, caused diseases, led to its eventual demise.[123] Still, some resisted its abandonment.[124] For his part, Oliver Wendell Holmes (physician, 1809-1894), father of the famous jurist Oliver Wendell Holmes Jr, gave his candid view of the age-old therapy of bloodletting when he wrote: "The lancet was the magician's wand of the dark ages of medicine."[125]

In 1980, G.R. Seigworth, who had done much research on bloodletting, wrote: "It seems hard to believe that the many educated observers over the centuries were completely wrong in their assessment of clinical improvement following bloodletting."[126] Evidence has proven the practice to be futile in most cases. Ironically, what was sincerely thought to be a benevolent measure for the good of patients was often harmful to them. The maxim *Primum non nocere* was unwittingly violated.[127] Yet, even as the practice was criticized for being often useless, it persisted. Those who used it, countered in their defense: "We were governed by the best light we had; we thought we were right, and so we are justified."[128] As one author puts it: "(B)lind adherence to a therapeutic regimen can cause trouble, and so can the uncritical extension of a remedy from one disease to another, and so can the failure to critically evaluate any clinical

---

[123] As early as 1830, Pierre-Charles-Alexandre Louis (1787-1872) began documenting the course of diseases systematically and how they responded to treatment. His studies showed by statistical proof the uselessness of bloodletting in the treatment of pneumonia. See Garrison, An Introduction to the History of Medicine, *supra* note 94, 411. By the nineteenth century, bloodletting was being severely criticized. See G. R. Seigworth, "Bloodletting Over the Centuries," *supra* note 110, 2024.

[124] Flint, Practice of Medicine, 133. The author states: "It can hardly be doubted that this measure was formerly adopted too indiscriminately, and often employed too largely, but the natural tendency being to pass from one extreme to another, the utility of bloodletting in certain cases, at the present time, is perhaps not sufficiently appreciated." See also Risse, "The Renaissance of Bloodletting: A Chapter in Modern Therapeutics," 3.

[125] Garrison, "The History of Bloodletting," *supra* note 92, 500.

[126] Seigworth, "Bloodletting Over the Centuries," *supra* note 110, 2027.

[127] "Above all [or first] do no harm." This maxim calls to mind the Hippocratic oath: "I will apply dietetic measure for the benefit of the sick according to my ability and judgment; I will keep them from harm and injustice." Translated by Ludwig Edelstein in The Hippocratic Oath at http://www.med.virginia.edu/hs-library/historical/antiqua/texto.htm.

[128] Estes, "George Washington and the Doctors: Treating America's First Superhero," *supra* note 91, 43-57.

improvement in relation to the remedy. ... The devotees of bloodletting sinned in all three respects."[129]

Was the longevity of such a useless therapy as bloodletting simply the result of ignorance, or was it also a question of control and paternalism? The answer may best be supplied by Garrison, who makes the following comment: "History teaches everywhere that permanent ignorance and superstition are the results of the oppression of mankind by fanatical overmen. In medicine, this is sometimes ludicrously true."[130]

These were times when, in the name of the 'life is sacred' principle, the blind determination of doctors to save lives, at all costs, often resulted in premature death or sickness. However, these were also times when the patient had little to say about the treatment to be administered, he was at the mercy of the physician.

The advent of blood transfusion

While bloodletting continued as a standard medical procedure even in the face of criticism, other uses for blood were being considered. Among the miraculous properties assigned to blood, considered the 'bearer of life,' was its power to rejuvenate. Blood baths were thought by some to help regain youth and vigor.[131] It was not a difficult leap to think of introducing young blood into the veins of an aging person in an attempt to help him rejuvenate. Though some believed that blood transfusions were practiced as far back as the ancient Egyptians,[132] the earliest record of such an attempt is reported to be in 1492 when

---

[129] King, Medical Thinking – A Historical Preface, 242-3.

[130] Garrison, An Introduction to the History of Medicine, *supra* note 94.

[131] Héritier, La sève de l'homme, *supra* note 102, 11, where reference is made to the countess Erzebeth Bathory of Hungary (16th century), who is said to have sacrificed six hundred young virgins to bathe in their blood.

[132] Penmery, Les origines de la transfusion sanguine, *infra* note 134, 57.

Pope Innocent VIII was purported to have been given the blood of three young men. It is not known exactly how the blood may have been administered, but it was to be to no avail, since the Pope died and, in the process, so did the three young men. The doctor, for his part, fled.[133] During this period of the Middle Ages reference is made to transfusing blood to humans, but there are no specific accounts of any transfusion having been actually carried out.[134]

It was not until 1628, when William Harvey's (English physician, 1578-1657) discovery of the circulation of blood gave a new direction to medicine, that blood transfusion experimentation began in earnest. Until then, the Galenic physiology taught that there were two types of blood, the venous and the arterial, each having different pathways and functions. According to this concept, blood, believed to be produced by the liver,[135] ebbed and flowed through arteries and veins and sloshed through imagined pores in the heart.[136] Harvey's research

---

133 Houdre, Aperçu sur l'historique de la transfusion sanguine depuis les origines jusqu'au XIXème siècle (Thèse pour le doctorat en médecine), 8. There is controversy as to whether this account is accurate or not. See the exchange of correspondence on this matter in "Correspondence," 553-4, 633. See also Lindeboom, "The story of a blood transfusion to a pope," 455.

134 Penmery, Les origines de la transfusion sanguine, 2. One quote from the 15th century stated:

> "Et pourquoi nos vieillards aussi qui sont destitués de toute aide ne suceront-ils le lait d'une jeune fille? Et le sang d'un jeune adolescent, qui le veuille bien, qui soit sain, gai, tempéré, qui ait le sang fort bon et par aventure trop en abondance? Qu'ils le sucent donc à la façon des airondes de la veine du bras gauche ouverte jusques à une ou deux onces."

Another quote from the 16th century stated:

> "Que l'on prenne un robuste jeune homme, en bonne santé et plein de sang vigoureux; que l'on tienne auprès de lui un autre, épuisé de toutes forces, maigre, décharné et à la respiration haletante; que l'homme de l'art ait des tuyaux d'argent s'adaptant les uns aux autres; qu'il ouvre une artère du sujet robuste, y insère un tuyau et l'y maintienne; qu'il ouvre immédiatement une artère du malade et y insère l'autre tuyau; ensuite qu'il ajuste les deux tuyaux ensemble et qu'il laisse le sang du sujet en bonne santé s'élancer, chaud et vigoureux, dans le malade, apporter la source de vie et chasser toute la faiblesse. "

135 This belief can be traced back to the Sumerians for whom "the liver, as the source of blood, was regarded as the seat of the soul." Garrison, An Introduction to the History of Medicine, *supra* note 94, 63.

136 Porter, The Greatest Benefit to Mankind, *supra* note 107, 211-6. Harvey described the circulation of blood in the following manner (at 214):

> "Since all things, both argument and ocular demonstration, show that the blood passes through the lungs and heart by the force of the ventricles, and is sent for distribution to all parts of the body, where it makes its way into the veins and porosities of the flesh, and then flows by the veins from the circumference on every side to the center, from the lesser to the greater veins, and is by them finally

clearly disproved this. His experimental methods, which included measuring flow and volume, helped to conceptualize the body mechanically instead of mystically. He did, however, continue to believe that the body was moved by vital forces.

Some of Harvey's colleagues, impressed by his research on circulation, carried on their own research with blood. In particular, Christopher Wren (English architect, 1632-1723) and Robert Boyle (English chemist, 1627-1691) reported on the effects of infusing different substances, such as opium, into the blood stream of both animals and humans.[137] A French Benedictine monk, Dom Robert des Gabets, is credited with being the first to propose the idea of performing a blood transfusion on an animal or a human in 1658.[138] However, Richard Lower (English physician and anatomist, 1631-1691), carried out the first recorded transfusion on an animal in February 1665.[139] This successful experiment (it was considered a success because the dog who received the blood did not die; the donor dog however bled to death) moved researchers to envision endless possibilities for this new therapy. 'Would a fierce dog become tame by being stocked with the blood of a cowardly dog or would the recipient's fur color change to that of the donor?' asked Boyle.[140]

French physician and ardent defender of blood transfusion therapy, Jean-

---

discharged into the vena cava and right auricle of the heart, and this in such a quantity or in such a flux and reflux thither by the arteries, hither by the veins, as cannot possibly be supplied by purposes of nutrition; it is absolutely necessary to conclude that the blood in the animal body is impelled in a circle, and is in a state of ceaseless motion."

137 Penmery, Les origines de la transfusion sanguine, *supra* note 134, 5, 6.

138 Penmery, Les origines de la transfusion sanguine, *supra* note 134, 13-14. Jean-Baptiste Denis claimed that Dom Robert des Gabets was the first to propose the idea of blood transfusion as a therapy. Richard Lower contested this, claiming that he was the first to conceive this idea. He had, in effect, carried out transfusions on animals as early as 1665, 15.

139 Penmery, Les origines de la transfusion sanguine, *supra* note 134, 15-6. According to Garrison, An Introduction to the History of Medicine, *supra* note 94, 273: "J.D. Major (1662), Caspar Scotus (1664), Elsholtz (*Clysmata nova*, 1665) made the first successful intravenous injections in man. Major published his *Chirurgia infusoria* at Kiel in 1667. Priority in transfusion has been claimed for Francesco Folli (1654), but the first authenticated records are those of R. Lower (1665-1667) and A. Coga (1667)."

140 Starr, Blood, An Epic History of Medicine and Commerce, *supra* note 115, 9.

Baptiste Denis (approx. 1635-1704), reasoned that since blood lost through bloodletting needed to be replaced, why not replace it with blood through a transfusion. For those opposed to phlebotomy he argued that since it was believed that 'corrupted' blood was present for all sickness, a transfusion would be the ideal way to purify the blood.[141] In this fashion, he hoped to convince both proponents and opponents of bloodletting of the value of blood transfusion therapy. Instead of transfusing human blood, Denis favored animal blood since he believed it was not corrupted with human vices and moods.[142] Denis believed that, as with bloodletting, blood transfusion would heal most disorders: pleurisy, small pox, leprosy, cancers, ulcers, epilepsy, madness, as well as most illnesses arising from what he believed to be 'corrupted' blood.[143]

On 15 June 1667, Denis practiced the first recorded transfusion on a human. Using the blood of a sheep, he transfused approximately 270 grams of blood into the veins of a teenage boy suffering from a severe fever resulting from copious bloodletting. According to Denis' observations, the transfusion was a success since the young man recovered and eventually regained his health.[144] In England, Lower followed suit on 23 November 1667, by transfusing sheep's blood into a thirty-two year old man named Arthur Coga, who was suffering from insanity. Again, as was the case with Denis, the transfusion was considered a success because the patient did not die. Others attempted transfusions in Germany, Holland and Italy, making exaggerated claims as to the results obtained.[145]

During the summer of 1667, Denis unsuccessfully transfused a Swedish nobleman. Later the same year, a 34-year-old man, Antoine Mauroy, who had been suffering from mental illness for several years, was brought to Denis.

---

[141] Penmery, Les origines de la transfusion sanguine, *supra* note 134, 32.

[142] *Ibid.*, 33.

[143] *Ibid.*

[144] *Ibid.*, 34-5.

[145] Starr, Blood, An Epic History of Medicine and Commerce, *supra* note 115, 12.

Mauroy had been bled many times to treat his attacks of insanity. Finally, Denis transfused him with five or six ounces of blood from a calf, carrying out the procedure before a large crowd of spectators. Mauroy 'improved' slightly, so Denis decided to give him a second transfusion of an even larger amount of blood (approx. 1 lb.). He improved sufficiently for the transfusion to be considered a success. On 10 February 1668, Denis transfused a partially paralyzed woman who survived for a short time. Mauroy, in the meantime, was again having continued bouts of lunacy, and was brought back by his wife, Périne, to Denis for an additional blood transfusion. A third transfusion was attempted, but could not be carried out because of the patient's convulsions. Mauroy died, and a lawsuit followed. Périne, who was supported by doctors who strongly opposed blood transfusions, accused Denis of causing the death of her husband. Denis countered by filing a complaint against the doctors involved with Périne, and by accusing her of poisoning Mauroy. Denis was not convicted, but the negative publicity surrounding the lawsuit resulted in a ban, in 1670, by the Parliament of Paris on any further transfusions.[146] Now considered dangerous and inefficient, transfusions fell into disrepute for the next 150 years.

Despite the existence of earlier claims,[147] the first credible report of a man to man blood transfusion came in 1818, from James Blundell (1790-1877).[148] After carrying out systematic and extensive experiments with animal transfusion,

---

[146] Penmery, Les origines de la transfusion sanguine, *supra* note 134, 63-71. Regarding the order of the Parliament of Paris, Penmery quotes Dictionnaire des arrêtes, de Brillon (1717): "Défense à tout Médecins et Chirurgiens d'exercer la transfusion du sang, à peine de punition corporelle. Arrêt du P. de Paris du 10 janvier 1670 Journal des Adu. Tom. 3. Liv. 10. Ch. 15. Les épreuves extraordinaires sont ordinairement dangereuses; et, pour une qui réussit, toutes les autres deviennent mortelles."

[147] For example, in 1667, Claude Tardy, a Parisian doctor, referring to material he taught 13 years earlier at the Faculté de Médecine de Paris, published two documents in which he described and illustrated man-to-man blood transfusions. However, authors in the next century dismissed his accounts as too simplistic which could only be the fruit of his imagination. See Penmery, Les origines de la transfusion sanguine, *supra* note 134, 49-51.

[148] Blundell, "Experiments on the Transfusion of Blood by the Syringe," 56; Blundell, "Some account of a case of obstinate vomiting in which an attempt was made to prolong life by the injection of blood into the veins," 310.

Blundell concluded, "the blood of animals might ... be harmful to human beings."[149] By the end of the nineteenth century, "the use of animal blood was abandoned for human transfusion therapy."[150] Favoring the use of human blood, Blundell transfused ten patients over a period of eleven years; five patients survived.[151] Blundell was acting on the belief that blood was "alive" and that past failures in transfusion practice were mainly due to technical details. He developed a variety of apparatus that he believed did not cause blood to lose "its life-giving properties." He was also probably the first to use the syringe in transfusion.[152] Some members of the Medical Society of London were opposed to these transfusions. They believed that a patient who survived a transfusion would have recovered regardless. A study in 1849 reviewed 48 reported cases of transfusions, of which 18 resulted in the death of the patient.[153] Several years later in the mid-1800s, English surgeon Alfred Higginson is reported to have performed transfusions on seven patients, five of whom died.[154] In the United States, various attempts were made at transfusion therapy during this time. The earliest recorded successful attempt was in 1795 by a Dr Philip Syng Physic (1768-1837) of Philadelphia. Transfusions were also reported in Annapolis in 1849, in New Orleans in 1858, and on four occasions by the Union Army during the Civil War.[155]

---

[149] Hagen, "Blood: Gift or Merchandise," 11:12.

[150] Soloman, III American Association of Blood Banks Administrative Manual, 1.

[151] Jones, "The Influence of James Blundell on the Development of Blood Transfusion," 242, 244-7.

[152] Jones, "The Influence of James Blundell on the Development of Blood Transfusion," *supra* note 151, 244-7. See also McClure, "Transfusion of Blood," 99. According to this article, Blundell's use of the syringe was limited to one, thus very little blood could be transfused through this method. Professor H. von Zeimssen, Director of the Medical Clinic in Munich, in 1892, developed a method using several syringes where he could transfuse an average of 300 cc. of blood.

[153] Routh, "Remarks Statistical and General on Transfusion of Blood," 114.

[154] Higginson, "Report of Seven Cases of Transfusion of Blood, With a Description of the Instrument Invented by the Author," 102-10 quoted in Starr, Blood, An Epic History of Medicine and Commerce, *supra* note 115, 38.

[155] Schmidt, "Transfusion in America in the Eighteenth and Nineteenth Centuries," 1319-20; Rutkow, American Surgery, An Illustrated History, 146-7.

While transfusions were becoming popular across Europe, as with earlier efforts these were generally not very successful. One Polish doctor's statistical research in 1873 showed that 56 percent of transfusions ended in death.[156] Because of the suffering and the mortality associated with transfusions, the practice again fell into disrepute. More research would be necessary to understand the nature of blood which we now know to be a complex heterogeneous tissue composed of several elements such as lymphocytes, monocytes, platelets, eosinophils, basophils, and plasma.[157]

Karl Landsteiner (1868-1943), considered the "father of blood groups,"[158] led the way in this research with the discovery of blood groups in 1901.[159] Alexis Carrel (1873-1944) developed a direct end-to-end suture of blood vessels known as vascular anastomosis.[160] To show the importance of cross matching, American physician, Reuben Ottenberg, relying on Landsteiner's research, carried on a five year study at Mount Sinai Hospital on pretransfusion testing.[161] However, even after these discoveries blood transfusion was still not widely used by doctors, that is, until the advent of the First World War.

"War is good for medicine" wrote one author.[162] This was to prove true for blood transfusion. During the course of the majors wars of the twentieth century, with blood flowing in unprecedented quantities, transfusion therapy developed

---

[156] Starr, Blood, An Epic History of Medicine and Commerce, *supra* note 115, 38.

[157] According to one author, Titmuss, The Gift Relationship, 247, one drop of blood is said to contain 250,000 red corpuscles, 400,000 white corpuscles and 15,000,000 platelets.

[158] Fleming, Medical Milestones, 188.

[159] Oberman, Clinical Practice of Transfusion Medicine, 24. See also Rossi, Simon & Moss, Principles of Transfusion Medicine, 6. Though the full impact of his discovery was not initially understood, his work is described as "a burst of light in a darkened room. He gave us our first glimpse of immunohematology and transplantation biology and provided the tools for important discoveries in genetics, anthropology, and forensic medicine."

[160] Rossi, Simon & Moss, Principles of Transfusion Medicine, *supra* note 159, 6.

[161] Ottenberg, "Accidents in Transfusion," 2138-40.

[162] Porter, The Greatest Benefit to Mankind, *supra* note 107, 652.

into the standard medical practice it is today. It would replace bloodletting as the "queen of remedies"; and many would eventually come to believe that "modern medicine could not survive without it."[163] Doctors on both sides worked frantically to save the lives of those injured by the enemy, transfusing more and more blood as the conflicts became larger and deadlier. This development of blood transfusion therapy throughout the wars of the 20th century is well summarized by P. Ellis as follows:

World War I:

-The ABO blood group had been discovered (1900) and was now used as a basis for selecting donors.

-The "universal donor" concept had been formulated by Ottenberg (1911).

-Anticoagulant was first used on a widespread basis.

-Pretransfusion testing was not routinely performed.

-Donor criteria were developed.

-Widespread use of plasma began.

Spanish Civil War:

-Blood was drawn from civilians for the benefit of war casualties.

-Criteria for transfusion were developed.

-Hemorrhage was treated with red blood cells.

-Shock was treated with plasma.

World War II:

-Blood was drawn in a closed system.

-Much information was gathered on the treatment of shock.

-Blood was airlifted from the United States for use overseas

163 Masson, History of the Blood Transfusion Service in Edinburgh, 92.

instead of being drawn locally.

-Hemolysin testing was performed on type O blood.

-Low titered Os were used as universal donors.

-It was found that blood could be transported without being hemolyzed.

-The shelf life of blood was extended to as long as seven weeks without reported ill effects.

-Autotransfusion was used when blood was in "short-supply."

-Packed red blood cells were widely used.

-Filters were used for plasma infusions.

-Fresh frozen plasma (FFP) received some limited use. It was, however, difficult to store at the front lines.

-Transfusion-related hepatitis was discovered.

Korean War:

-In organized collection, donors were typed at the collection site and only type Os were drawn.

-A closed system (bottle) with acid citrate dextrose (ACD) was used for collection.

-A central reporting program for reporting post-transfusion hepatitis was implemented.

-Methods for sterilizing plasma were attempted.

-Storage and transportation studies were conducted–as storage at room temperature was found to cause irreversible damage.

Vietnam War:

-A high risk of hepatitis was found in Vietnam; hence, residents and soldiers there were not good donors.

-There was also a high risk of malaria and syphilis in

Vietnam.

-Blood was drawn in Japan and shipped to Vietnam.

-Blood was kept for 31 days.

-Work was conducted on ACD-adenine.[164]

Staggering quantities of donated blood were sent to the battlefield during some of these wars.[165] Researchers were frantically looking for ways to meet the demands imposed on health facilities by modern warfare. New methods for harvesting and storing blood were developed. Even cadavers became a potential source of blood.[166] In Canada, the Red Cross established its first blood donor clinic in January 1940. Later that same year, Charles H. Best (physiologist, 1899-1978), with financing from the Canadian Ministry of Defense, succeeded in developing a method of reducing plasma serum to powder. Connaught Laboratories produced the 'miracle' powder and the Red Cross entered the business of distributing it to the front.[167] Connaught would stay in the blood business until June 1987, when its credibility was seriously tarnished by the blood scandal of the 1980s. In the United States, Edwin Joseph Cohn (biochemist, 1892-1953), devised methods of producing human plasma fractions such as serum albumin, gamma globulin, fibrinogen, and fibrin, which were used for treating the

---

[164] This table appears in an article by Ellis, Transfusion Therapy, Principles and Procedures, 5. For a first-hand account of a surgeon's experience with blood transfusion during both World Wars see: Guiou, Transfusion, A Canadian Surgeon's Story in War and in Peace.

[165] Approximately 2.5 million donations were made during the course of World War II according to Picard, The Gift of Death, *infra* note 167, 26. Another author, referring to reports from the American Red Cross, mentions that by the end of 1943, the military had received "more than two and half million packages of dried plasma and nearly 125,000 ampoules of albumin." However, these would prove insufficient. See Starr, Blood, An Epic History of Medicine and Commerce, *supra* note 115, 121.

[166] McCullough, Transfusion Medicine, 5.

[167] Picard, The Gift of Death, 20-2. Colonel Albert E. Gooderham, himself involved in Red Cross activities, established Connaught Laboratories. Together, the Red Cross and Connaught Laboratories worked closely together to gather blood, process it, and send it to the front. During World War II, Connaught Laboratories produced a total of 436,000 bottles of dried plasma. During the last twelve months of the war, Canadians gave 890,000 blood donations, m ore than a third of all donations made during the war.

armed forces and later in civilian medicine.[168]

Normally, new products or drugs are introduced into medicine only after rigorous clinical trials to establish the risk/benefit factors. If the risks outweigh the benefits, the product is not approved. This procedure, however, was never followed with blood transfusions. In fact, according to the United States Congress' Office of Technology Assessment Task Force "data by which to evaluate the overall appropriate use of blood products do not exist."[169] There are no records of "randomized controlled trial(s)" establishing scientific proof of the benefits of blood transfusions.[170] Nevertheless, blood transfusion did become standard procedure. Since patients were surviving, the therapy was deemed to be beneficial.

Bloodletting took on a new meaning – no longer was it practiced for therapeutic reasons as it had been for millenniums – the donor was now being asked to voluntarily give up part of his precious blood for an unknown patient.[171] Donating blood to the Red Cross was considered a patriotic duty.[172] The blood industry developed into a prosperous business. In North America, for example, blood was being separated, processed, freeze-dried, bagged and shipped to hospitals locally and in different parts of the world. Blood banks were established and the public was admonished to give 'the gift of life.' In the United States the

---

168 "Cohn, Edwin Joseph" Encyclopaedia Britannica Online http://members.eb.com/bol/topic?eu=25072&sctn=1&pm=1 [Accessed 26 April 1999].

169 U.S Congress, Office of Technology Assessment Task Force, Blood Technologies, Services, and Issues, 121.

170 Spence, Blood and Blood Products: Safety and Risk, 83.

171 Mollison, Engelfriet & Contreras, Blood Transfusion in Clinical Medicine, 1. Surprisingly, in this textbook the authors are of the view that bloodletting was harmless, even citing Benjamin Rush's work as an example. It goes on to state that bloodletting "has come back into fashion although in the more sophisticated form of plasma or red cell exchange."

172 During the First World War, "the American Red Cross distributed a poster of the Stars and Stripes alongside the Red Cross flag with the slogan 'Loyalty to one means loyalty to both.'" This loyalty extended to donating blood since during the Second World War, the Red Cross was instrumental in collecting blood in support of the war effort. See Picard, The Gift of Death, *supra* note 167, 20.

practice of collecting blood took on gigantic proportions: in 1992 alone a staggering 13,588,000 units were collected.[173] With the development of plasmapheresis, the harvest of raw plasma became a thriving business, both for the donor, from whom the plasma was bought, and for the collection agency that would resell it for a handsome profit. Since only plasma was collected, the red cells being re-infused in the donor, it was possible to harvest from the same individual as often as twice a week or 104 times a year. Those with rare blood types or immunity factors could sell for a higher price. In one case, it is reported that a woman earned more than $80,000 a year selling her blood.[174] The unemployed, the indigent, the substance-addicted, and even prisoners saw an opportunity for extra income.

Thus, during the last quarter century, blood banking and transfusion medicine developed into a complex, sophisticated, medical-technical discipline.[175] However, the procedure became so commonplace that physicians gave little thought to the complexity of blood and its uniqueness in each individual.[176] In fact, to this day "clinicians administer blood without giving much thought to the indications for its use, the proper dose required, and the potential adverse consequences."[177] With approximately 14 million units of blood being transfused

---

[173] McCullough, Transfusion Medicine, *supra* note 166, 19.

[174] *U.S. v. Garber*, 589 F. 2d 843, 845 (5th Cir. 1979).

[175] For a detailed explanation of the preparation and administration of blood products see: Calhoune, Clinical Practice of Transfusion Medicine, 305-33.

[176] Miller, Transfusion Therapy, Principles and Procedures, *supra* note 164, 295. According to this author: "Blood transfusion has become so commonplace that the unique nature of this form of therapy is often overlooked. Transfusionists must remember that the transfusion process is a special kind of transplant, with the transfer of living tissue from one person to another. Furthermore, blood is a highly complex, heterogeneous tissue, much more so than most people realize. Besides erythrocytes (which have over 350 blood groups distinguishing one individual from another), there are lymphocytes, monocytes, platelets, eosinophils, basophils, and plasma with essential nutrients, wastes, immunoglobulins, transport proteins, and a potpourri of clotting proteins. Not only is blood unique to each individual, but the transfusion process (collection, long-term storage and reinfusion) carries with it a variety of special problems and risks…."

[177] Kevy & Gorlin, Hematology of Infancy and Childhood, 1786.

in just one year in the United States alone, problems were sure to develop.[178]

The AIDS crisis jolted both health professionals and the public into awareness of the potential dangers associated with blood. However, that the "risks of transfusion are legion" was well known even before the crisis.[179] Warnings about the dangers of transfusion-transmitted hepatitis were being sounded as early as 1943.[180] That year, thousands of bottles of dried plasma from Canada had to be destroyed when soldiers contracted a bacterial infection in a tainted-blood problem that received little publicity.[181] In 1948, Dr Capps pointed to research which indicated that as many as 20% of patients were being infected by hepatitis from contaminated blood.[182] The problem, he pointed out, was compounded in the case of pooled blood.[183] In 1961, "the annual mortality from only 3 complications of blood transfusion (hemolytic reactions, overload and serum hepatitis) is computed to be 16,500" in the U.S.A. alone.[184] A later study found the occurrence of Non-A Non-B Hepatitis, due to contaminated blood, to be as high as 33%.[185] In 1965, Dr Louis Diamond, deploring the lack of proper training in transfusion practices wrote, "blood is often used wastefully, improperly, and dangerously."[186] Investigations revealed that possibly 'only 1%

---

[178] Rossi, Simon & Moss, Principles of Transfusion Medicine, *supra* note 159, 9.

[179] Miller, Transfusion Therapy, Principles and Procedures, *supra* note 164, 295. See also Mollison, Engelfriet & Contreras, Blood Transfusion in Clinical Medicine, *supra* note 171, xvii. The preface to this edition points out that in the first edition of the volume, 40 years earlier, only four pages were devoted to the subject of ill effects of transfusion. In the 9th edition, however, the longest chapter is devoted to infectious agents transmitted by transfusion.

[180] Beeson, "Jaundice Occurring One to Four Months After Transfusion of Blood or Plasma," 1332.

[181] Picard, The Gift of Death, *supra* note 167, 25.

[182] "Dangers of Blood Transfusion," Awake!, *supra* note 83. In 1966, Creutzfeldt found the incident to be as high as 28.6% in patients with more than 10 transfusions. See Gruber, Blood Replacement, 24.

[183] "Dangers of Blood Transfusion," *Ibid.*

[184] Wilson, Complications in Surgery and Their Management, 80.

[185] Stevens, "The Epidemiology of Non-A Non-B Hepatitis in the United States," 44: "Incidence rates ranged between 7 and 16 percent among recipients of blood from volunteer donors and up to 33 percent among recipients of blood from paid donors."

of transfusions were given on vital indication'.[187] Authors warned about 'over-enthusiastic transfusionists' who were administering needless transfusions; still others compared this reckless practice to playing "Russian roulette with bottles of blood" which resulted in thousands dying needlessly.[188]

Eventually, due to ensuing lawsuits, it became necessary for the medical community in the U.S.A. to convince state legislatures to adopt blood "shield" laws which defined blood and blood products as a service and not a product, thereby carrying no implied warranty. This, they hoped, would protect them from liability in cases of tainted blood products. This categorization of blood has been followed by other countries, thereby relieving hospitals, blood banks, and the Red Cross, from liability in cases of contaminated blood, except where negligence is proven.[189]

Significantly, evidence of the dangers associated with blood transfusion

---

186 Diamond, "History of Blood Banking in the United States," 42.

187 Gruber, Blood Replacement, *supra* note 182, 19: This manual on blood transfusion stated that from retrospective investigations, it was assumed that "35% to 50% of all transfusions are unnecessary and that only 1% are given on vital indication." In 1957, Dr Bruce Chown guessed that not 1% of transfusions been had been life-saving. See Chown, "Transfusions are Dangerous," 1037.

188 Zeitlin, "Warning on Over-Free use of Blood Transfusions," author states that in England about 200 died as a result of transfusions. He criticizes what he calls 'cosmetic' transfusions "which are performed more for the benefit of the relatives and the peace of mind of the doctor than for the well-being of the patient;" Crosby, "Misuse of Blood Transfusions," 1200. About the "thoughtless prescription of blood transfusion," the author writes "While the odds are in the physician's favor that nothing will go wrong, the patient takes the risk.;" Greenwalt estimated that blood transfusion contributed to at least 1,700 deaths annually in the United States with the morbidity rate being many times higher. In 1960, the chief legal adviser of the American Medical Association, B. D. Hirsh, was of the view that approximately 3,000 persons died annually in the USA from blood transfusions. See Gruber, Blood Replacement, *supra* note 182, 20-1. In Unger, "Medical-Legal Aspects of Blood Transfusion," 237: The author warns "Blood is dynamite! It can do a great deal of good or a great deal of harm. The mortality from blood transfusion equals that from either anesthesia or appendectomy. There is said to be approximately one death in 1,000 to 3,000 or possibly 5,000 transfusions. In the London area there has been reported one death for every 13,000 bottles of blood transfused." He goes on to add: "When one considers the vast number of patients transfused, the wonder is not that catastrophes occur but that they do not occur more often."

189 For example, in the Canadian case of *Pittman v. Bain*, [1994] 19 C.C.L.T. (2d) 1 (Ont. Ct. Gen. Div.) 1 at 99, the trial judge was of the view that "blood is not a manufactured product in the nature of other equipment and supplies, it is not, in my view, reasonable to imply a term that the Hospital, absent negligence on its part, warranted that it would be free of disease."

"was largely ignored by the medical profession as a whole."[190] This is surprising considering that there exists "no randomized controlled trial" from which proof of the benefit of blood transfusion could be found.[191] According to one physician "if one approached regulatory authorities today with a new product having the safety profile of human red cells, it probably would not be approved for clinical use."[192] Certain practices, adopted and maintained for decades by the medical community, such as the "transfusion trigger," have been described as being "cloaked in traditions, shrouded in obscurity, and unsubstantiated by clinical or experimental evidence."[193] In fact, even though transfusion medicine has become a daily part of the physicians' practice, "(t)here is a surprising, even appalling, lack of adequate studies on the value of, and indications for, the blood products in question."[194] As the procedure developed, over the years it became evident that there were "wide variations in transfusion practices", these practices often being

---

[190] Baron, "Blood, Sin, and Death: Jehovah's Witnesses and the American Patients' Rights Movement," 115.

[191] Spence, "Beneficial Aspects of Surgical Transfusion," Blood and Blood Products: Safety and Risk, *supra* note 170, 83.

[192] Picard, "Tragedy prompts bloodless solutions," A1. Comments by Robert Winslow, professor of Medicine at the University of California at San Diego during presentation "Is There A Potential Need for Blood Substitutes in Civilian and Noncivilian Situations?" (Address to the IV International Symposium on Blood Substitutes, 20 August 1991).

[193] Zauder, "How Did We Get a "Magic Number" for Preoperative Hematocrit/Hemoglobin Level?". Reporting in The Lancet on a Consensus Conference of the Royal College of Physicians at Edinburgh in May 1994, the author stated: "Despite more than 5 decades of established practice, doctors still do not agree about precisely when and why they should transfuse red cells and how efficacy can be assessed. … One message was clear, the traditional transfusion trigger – i.e., the critical haemoglobin value justifying transfusion intervention – needs to be considerably revised. … And despite the diversity of views, there was little dissension from the idea that a therapy that costs so much … deserved to be put on an altogether more substantial scientific basis." Napier, "Towards More Rational Use of Red Cells," 1280.

[194] Ellison & Silberstein, "A Commentary on Three Consensus Development Conferences on Transfusion Medicine," 624. According to the United States Congress' Office of Technology Assessment Task Force, "data by which to evaluate the overall appropriate use of blood products do not exist, in many cases because of lack of scientific precision concerning when a component or derivative should be administered." U.S Congress, Office of Technology Assessment Task Force, Blood Technologies, Services, and Issues, *supra* note 169, 121.

"based on habit rather than scientific data."[195] Even today, after "more than 5 decades of established practice, doctors still do not agree about precisely when and why they should transfuse red cells."[196] The uncertainty seems to exist because, as one survey found, "(d)efficiencies in knowledge of transfusion indications were widespread." The practice based on this lack of scientific research and reliance on "anecdotal information"[197] is passed on from chief resident to assistant resident and on to interns and medical students. As a result, it has been observed that "many physicians enter their definitive careers with a shallow and narrow understanding of the appropriate management of one of their most important therapeutic tools."[198]

However, since retrospective data and anecdotal information indicated that many more patients were surviving the procedure than were dying from it, and no doubt aided by "its reputation of mythical proportions,"[199] blood transfusion therapy remained 'the queen of remedies' with medical practitioners until, as we shall see, reports of the blood scandals of the 1980s began to appear in news headlines around the world.

Tainted blood episode

Of all the events surrounding modern blood transfusion therapy, the singular, most devastating one, which sounded the wakeup call to the dangers of transfused blood was, without a doubt, the tainted blood scandals of the 1980s.

---

[195] Stehling, "A Survey of Transfusion Practices Among Anesthesiologists," 61-2.

[196] Napier, "Towards More Rational use of Red Cells," *supra* note 193. The author also states that "For most areas of surgical practice the lack of incontrovertible proof of benefit from red-cell transfusion, despite subjective impressions, might seem disquieting. After all, what widely available drug could be used under such imprecise circumstances?"

[197] Thomson, "Blood Component Treatment: A Retrospective Audit in Five major London Hospitals," 734-6.

[198] Swisher & Petz, Clinical Practice of Transfusion Medicine, 4.

[199] Picard, "Tragedy Prompts Bloodless Solutions," *supra* note 192, A8.

For many, the "gift of life" became the "gift of death."[200] Populations all over the world were jolted into the realization that those who had received blood transfusions during the 1980s had been "unwitting participants in the lottery of death."[201] The stupor heightened as notification was sent out to millions of former blood transfusion recipients, advising them that they were at risk of having contacted AIDS and Hepatitis C.

Serious warnings of the possibility of AIDS being transmitted through blood transfusions started to surface in the U.S. in 1982.[202] In 1983, high-risk donor groups were identified and attempts were made to stop collecting blood from them.[203] To illustrate the danger of contamination from these high-risk groups, the example of Christopher Whitfield of Texas, a transient gay man who died of AIDS in 1983, is cited. He had sold his blood 48 times between 1982 and 1983. During that time he had no visible symptoms of AIDS and he lied when asked if he belonged to a high-risk group. His plasma had infected 65,000 doses of blood clotting agents that were distributed to 14 countries worldwide, including Canada, France, Jordan and Israel.[204] In 1984, an American study reported on 28 AIDS cases where the sole risk factor was blood transfusion.[205] Recognizing the danger of contamination from blood harvested from commercial donors, the Council of Ministers of the Council of Europe recommended the elimination of such imports altogether.[206] Such warnings were largely ignored by countries like

---

[200] For a detailed account of the events surrounding the Canadian tainted blood scandal see: Picard, The Gift of Death, *supra* note 167; McDuff, Le sang qui tue.

[201] Picard, The Gift of Death, *supra* note 167, 1.

[202] Institute of Medicine, HIV and the Blood Supply: An Analysis of Critical Decision-making, III-9.

[203] Picard, The Gift of Death, *supra* note 167, 72-3.

[204] ABC NEWS, 20/20 aired on 19 March 1987, hosts Hugh Downs & Barbara Walters, producer Joseph R. Lovett and correspondent Tom Jarriel; Starr, Blood, An Epic History of Medicine and Commerce, *supra* note 115, 293.

[205] Curran, "Acquired Immunodeficiency Syndrome (AIDS) Associated with Transfusions."

[206] Starr, Blood, An Epic History of Medicine and Commerce, *supra* note 115, 280.

England, Germany, France, Canada and Japan, who continued to rely heavily on what would later prove to be contaminated imported blood products, mostly from the U.S.[207] During the World Hemophilia Federation's annual meeting in June 1983, a Dutch representative, Cees Smit, whose research had helped Dutch authorities limit the importation of blood products, failed to convince the Federation to warn hemophiliacs of the impending danger.[208] As a result, hemophiliacs would become the group to suffer the most from tainted blood, with thousands dying. Yet, in spite of the growing number of warnings being sounded, the public in the United States and Canada was being reassured that the risk of contacting AIDS through blood products was only one in a million.[209]

One American doctor, D.R. Francis, candidly described the lack of response to these early warnings: "It was something like having a bend in the train track and sitting there and you hear the whistles and the signals are blinking and the tracks are beginning to shake, and they're saying, 'There's no train coming.'"[210]

The scandal then took on a more sinister, mercenary twist. After it became known that stocks of blood products were contaminated, in order to avoid heavy financial loses officials did not remove them from circulation.[211] In Canada, even

---

207 *Ibid.*, 278-92.

208 *Ibid.*, 282.

209 In Picard, The Gift of Death, *supra* note 167, 127, the footnote states: "The one-in-a-million risk, often cited over the years, seems to have come from a July 19, 1983 press conference where Dr. Roslyn Herst said, in response to a question, that the risk to transfusion recipients was one in a million. That figure was based on U.S. statistics that showed fourteen cases of transfusions AIDS over a three-year period during which there had been ten million transfusions." See also p. 64 which explains that in 1984, Health and Welfare in Canada distributed a pamphlet to the public stating that the risk was only two in a million. During that time, NACAIDS published a document to be inserted in *The Medical Post*, stating that there was "no conclusive proof" that AIDS could be transmitted through blood.

210 Quoted in Starr, Blood, An Epic History of Medicine and Commerce, *supra* note 115, 273 from Video deposition of Dr Donald R. Francis, 3 July 1992, District Court, Denver, Col., *Chris and Susie Quintana v. United Blood Services*, case no. 86CV11750 at 45.

211 Picard, The Gift of Death, *supra* note 167, 120; "Editorial," The Lancet, 1434: "It would be indefensible to allow prescription and home use of material known to at risk from HTLV III when apparently safer preparations are available."

after it was confirmed that untreated blood concentrates, such as Factor VIII, were potentially lethal, a concentrated effort was still made to distribute the remaining stocks even though safer, treated concentrates were now available, in inventory.[212] And, even when treated concentrates became available, they were initially only distributed to selected groups who found themselves to be on what would later come to be known to many hemophiliacs as a "Schindler's List."[213] In late 1984, despite being warned that a particular lot of concentrate contained plasma from three donors diagnosed with AIDS, the Canadian Red Cross made no attempts whatsoever to locate and destroy the lot.[214] Untreated blood products considered unsafe in one city were returned to the Red Cross warehouse in Ottawa, only to be redistributed to another area.[215] By using up their untreated stocks, the Canadian health system initially saved less than $2 million.[216] In return, more than 1,200 persons were infected with HIV and the Canadian government eventually had to pay out more than $1 billion in compensation.[217] After several years of investigations, criminal charges were eventually laid against the Red Cross Society, as well as against five doctors who occupied administrative positions in various organizations, for "criminal negligence and common nuisance by endangering the public."[218]

In France, health officials were brought to trial and sentenced to prison

---

[212] Picard, The Gift of Death, *supra* note 167, 119: "By May 1 (1985) the Red Cross had 7.8 millions units of heat-treated products in inventory, but during that month it delivered only 343,795 of those units to hemophilia treatment centers. Despite a healthy inventory and assurances that two large orders would arrive early in June, the priority lists were rigidly obeyed and the stock was held back so the unheated products could be used."

[213] *Ibid.*, 118.

[214] *Ibid.*, 117.

[215] *Ibid.*, 119.

[216] *Ibid.*, 198.

[217] Picard, "Blood Victims May See Cash by Year's End;" Thompson, Canada's tainted blood scandal: A timeline, CBC News Online, Nov. 20, 2002: cbc.ca/storyview/CBC/2002/11/20/blood_charges021120.

[218] *Ibid.*

terms and fines for having "knowingly distributed blood extracts contaminated with HIV."[219] One of these officials, former head of the National Blood Transfusion Centre, Dr Michel Garretta, was a major shareholder in one of the main suppliers of concentrate and had funneled more than $1 million to companies he controlled.[220] Even after it was well known that prisoners were a high-risk donor group, blood collected from French prisons continued to be used until late 1985, a practice which had been abandoned by several countries in the 1970s and early 1980s because of the threat of hepatitis.[221] In January 1985, even though they knew that blood supplies might be contaminated, French government officials delayed approving an American screening test for detecting HIV, to allow time for a domestic company to develop its own test. During the six month delay, patients were being infected.[222] Adding to the scandal, it was found that in 1985, after the French government had banned the use of untreated blood concentrates, 3.2 million of these potentially lethal units were nevertheless exported to West Germany, Italy, Spain, Portugal, Greece, Argentina, Iraq, Saudi Arabia, Egypt, Libya and Tunisia.[223] Through subsequent investigation, it also came to light that after banning the importation of U.S. blood concentrate, France was secretly importing plasma from third world 'vampire shops,' a dangerous practice followed by many other countries.[224] By using up their stock of untreated

---

219 "French Tainted Blood Affair Continues Beyond Court Sentence," 1047; Picard, "France makes an example of misdeeds." Dr Michel Garetta, former head of the National Blood Transfusion Centre, was condemned to four years in prison and a $100,000 fine. He was also ordered to pay about $3 million dollars in compensation to 70 victims. His former assistant, Dr Jean-Pierre Alain, was also sentenced to four years in prison (two years were suspended). Dr Jacques Roux, former Director General of Health, received a suspended sentence of four years.

220 Picard, The Gift of Death, *supra* note 167, 196, 199. Garretta's lawyer complained that his client was really a scapegoat in this scandal and compared him to the famous Jean-Baptiste Denis who, in 1668, was charged with murder in the death of his patient Antoine Mauroy following a blood transfusion.

221 Nau & Nouchi, "Fatal Attraction in Prisoners' Blood," 15; Starr, Blood, An Epic History of Medicine and Commerce, *supra* note 115, 315.

222 Patel, "France Faces Fresh HIV Blood Scandal," 7.

223 "New Scandal Erupts in France Over Export of Blood Products," 60.

224 Starr, Blood, An Epic History of Medicine and Commerce, *supra* note 115, 205.

blood concentrate and delaying testing, the French blood system saved a meager $4 million.[225] However, the results in human tragedy were staggering: "1 500 hemophiliacs were infected with HIV and at least 256 have since died of AIDS" (report dated 15 August 1992).[226]

Where countries responded quickly to the crisis, the consequences were less devastating. In Belgium, for example, only 7% of hemophiliacs were infected and in Sweden 16%. However, elsewhere the outcome was tragic. In Spain, 90% of hemophiliacs were infected,[227] in Denmark 64% and in England 32%.[228] Worldwide, over 40,000 hemophiliacs have tested positive for HIV.[229] For these victims, this was a real "Holocaust."[230]

Moreover, not only hemophiliacs were infected. All recipients of blood products were exposed to the lethal consequences of tainted blood. In the U.S., for example, while more than 8,000 hemophiliacs were infected, more than 12,000 other blood recipients were also infected from blood products.[231] Eventually, 22 countries, including most of Europe, Canada and Thailand established compensation funds. In the U.S., hemophiliacs were able to work out a compensation settlement with the industry worth $640 million.

Money and statistics cannot, however, accurately portray the toll of human suffering caused by the scandal. There are a few real life scenarios that help depict the depth of the agony: The mother explaining to her 11-year-old son that he has a fatal disease caused by a *teaspoon* of unnecessary blood administered to

---

225 Picard, The Gift of Death, *supra* note 167, 198.

226 "Prison Sentences for French Blood Transfusion Officials," 8.

227 Picard, The Gift of Death, *supra* note 167, 204.

228 Starr, Blood, An Epic History of Medicine and Commerce, *supra* note 115, 320.

229 *Ibid.*,346.

230 *Ibid.*, 343.

231 *Ibid.*, 337.

him as a baby.[232] Or, the lawyer explaining to a widow that her husband had been infected with HIV five years earlier, but the treating physician had decided, in a blush of paternalism, that his patient "was too emotionally fragile to be told of his transfusion of bad blood" – the wife had in turn been infected by the husband.[233] The pain of a mother and father, having to explain to their 11-year-old twins that they are going to die – unfortunately, the children had received some of the untreated blood products that were being liquidated, while treated products sat on the shelves.[234] The wife coping with emotional turmoil as she marks the months "with CD4 counts [a marker for the progression of AIDS]," watching and waiting for her husband to die.[235] The student facing the ostracism of being an HIV-positive child who is expelled from school and seeing his family driven from home and neighborhood.[236] For these individuals, blood held no mystic healing power; it was a merciless killer.

As tainted-blood scandals unfolded in different parts of the world, it became evident that HIV was not the only virus to infect patients who received blood products, though it was the most deadly.[237] It is now known that additional hundreds of thousands of blood product recipients worldwide were contaminated with Hepatitis C.[238] For example, in Canada, it was reported that as many as

---

232 Carlson, "Clients Living Proof of Canada's Tainted-Blood Scandal," 4.

233 This is one of the few cases where a victim of AIDS won a lawsuit against a physician. The judge, however, did not condemn the hospital, the doctor, and the Red Cross for using tainted blood. They were only held liable for failure to give timely notice to the patient and his family. See *Pittman Estate v. Bain*, *supra* note 189.

234 Picard, The Gift of Death, *supra* note 167, 121.

235 *Ibid.*, 180-1.

236 Starr, Blood, An Epic History of Medicine and Commerce, *supra* note 115, 316.

237 Is the Scandal Really Over? A report in 1993 accused France of pooling samples of blood to use fewer test kits. The practice is dangerous since it dilutes the HIV antibodies and can produce a false negative result. See Patel, "French 'Cut Corner' Over HIV Testing," 11. Another report told about a German licensed company that failed to test every blood donation separately, as required by law. Plasma which came from this company infected at least three patients. See MacKenzie, "How Safe is Europe's Blood?," 12.

238 Starr, Blood, An Epic History of Medicine and Commerce, *supra* note 115, 346.

60,000 had been infected.[239] Countries are still trying to tally the final number of victims and the amount of compensation to award them. In 1999, the Canadian government offered to set up a fund worth over $1,118,000,000 for persons infected with hepatitis C through blood transfusion received between 1986 and 1990.[240]

The risks associated to blood transfusion therapy are now widely known. Recent studies have shown that blood transfusion is "associated with a 35% greater risk of serious bacterial infection and a 52% greater risk of pneumonia."[241] Other studies indicate that blood transfusions "have a negative long-term impact … including increased risk of infections, complicated wound healing, and acceleration of local growth and/or dissemination of tumors" and should be viewed as "the transplantation of cellular and soluble elements and that they cause substantial alterations in the immune responsiveness of recipients."[242] As stated by one author, in view of the potentially lethal effects of blood products, these "should be considered potentially dangerous drugs."[243]

There is no doubt that transfusion therapy and unsafe medical practices during the tainted-blood episodes of the 1980s were indeed, in many cases, a "lottery of death" for the unwilling participants. This dreadful tale, which received extensive media coverage, helped doctors and patients to better understand that blood can be a dangerous product. Paternalism, or what was left

---

[239] Picard, "Krever Report Fallout Looks Devastating," A1: Results from the Krever Inquiry indicated that "at least 60,000 transfusions recipients contracted hepatitis C, a potentially debilitating liver disease."

[240] The Gazette (28 June 1999) A 14. Notice of proposed settlement was approved by Mr Justice Winkler of the Superior Court of Justice for Ontario, Mr Justice K. Smith of the Supreme Court of British Columbia and Madame Justice Morneau of the Superior Court of Quebec.

[241] Carson, "Risk of Bacterial Infection Associated with Allogeneic Blood Transfusion Among Patients Undergoing Hip Fracture Repair," 694.

[242] Grzelak, "Blood Transfusions Downregulate Hematopoiesis and Subsequently Downregulate the Immune Response," 1102. See also Vrielink & Reesink, "Transfusion – Transmissible Infections," 396.

[243] Fakhry & Sheldon, Textbook of Surgery, 118, 124-5.

of it, was dealt a crippling blow. From now on, patients would be asking questions that doctors would have to answer, also informing them of the risks associated with blood products. The media would be watching. The main players of the tainted-blood saga had been doctors, hospitals and agencies handling blood products, such as the Red Cross. As a result, the medical profession started being viewed more critically and more realistically, dropping a few notches from what Professor Baron called "the status of an established state church."[244] The spell had been broken.

Legal battles over the right of a patient to refuse blood

A survey of 28 different religious groups revealed that only Jehovah's Witnesses firmly object, for conscientious reasons, to the use of blood transfusion as medical therapy, while they accept other forms of standard medical treatment.[245] They have consistently taken this stand since 1945, at a time when blood transfusion was emerging as standard therapy. They maintained this position through the dark years of the tainted blood episode and continue to do so today. Their religious belief that blood transfusion violates God's law brought them into a head-on collision course with the medical profession's 'dogma' that blood is "the gift of life."

Initially, it would seem that the issue of medical decision-making by a competent adult was a straightforward matter. In an often quoted 1914 decision, American jurist Cardozo stated quite plainly that: "(e)very human being of adult years and sound mind has a right to determine what shall be done with his own body."[246] However, one must keep in mind that this was a time when biomedical ethics had not yet evolved; paternalism was strong and "the physician enjoyed

---

244 Baron, Blood, Sin, and Death: Jehovah's Witnesses and the American Patients' Rights Movement, *supra* note 190, 115.

245 Catholic Hospital Association, Religious Aspects of Medical Care: A Handbook of Religious Practices of All Faiths, 1-69.

autonomy and independence, alone with God and the patient, and alone with God, when deciding, in *loco parentis*, what was best for the patient.[247] It is not surprising that hospitals and physicians consistently, and often successfully, petitioned the courts to override the decision of a competent adult Jehovah's Witness patient refusing blood. In such a context, it took courage and determination to challenge the medical establishment both in courts and in the media, and claim the right to make autonomous medical decisions.[248]

In many of these cases, third party interests were invoked to override the patient's bodily self-determination, personal privacy and religious freedom. Notions such as "abandonment" of minor children or risk of liability for doctors and hospitals were considered.[249] In the U.S., the leading case on this issue was *In re President and Directors of Georgetown College, Inc.*,[250] in which Judge Skelly Wright ordered that blood transfusions be administered to Mrs Jesse Jones, who was *in extremis* following heavy bleeding from a ruptured ulcer. Mrs Jones and her husband had a seven month old son. Both parents were Jehovah's Witnesses and would not consent to blood transfusion.[251] After the president of Georgetown University, Father Bunn, pleaded to no avail with Mrs Jones that she changed her mind, hospital attorneys unsuccessfully petitioned a trial judge to

---

246 *Schloendorff v. Society of New York Hospital* (1914) 211 N. Y. 125.

247 Bendixen, "Preface" to Blood and Blood Products, xiii.

248 They were confronting the "American medical profession (which) had achieved something of the status of an established state church," and they were asking the courts to "take a neutral stance between the beliefs of their religion and those of American medicine. Baron, "Blood, Sin, and Death: Jehovah's Witnesses and the American Patients' Rights Movement," *supra* note 190.

249 The notion of 'abandonment' was considered in several cases. See for example: *Holmes v. Silver Cross Hosp.* 340 F. Supp. 125 (N.D. Ill 1972); *In re Osborne*, 294 A.2d 372 (D.C. 1972); *In re Brooks*, 32 Ill. 2d 361, 205 N.E.2d 435 (1965); *In re Melideo*, 88 Misc. 2d 974, 390 N.Y.S.2d 523 (Sup. Ct. 1976); *Fosmire v. Nicoleau*, 75 N.Y.2d 218, 551 N.E.2d 77, 551 N.Y.S.2d 876 (1990), 144 A.D.2d 8, 536 N.Y.S.2d 492 (1989); *Norwood Hospital v. Munoz*, 409 Mass.116, 564 N.E.2d 1017 (1991); *In re Dubreuil*, 629 So. 2d 819 (Fla. 1993), 603 So. 2d 538 (Fla. Dist. Ct. App. 1992).

250 331 F.2d 1000 (Wright, J., in chambers), 331 F.2d 1010 (D.C. Cir.) cert. denied, 377 U.S. 978 (1964).

251 *Ibid.*

override her refusal. The matter was then immediately brought before Justice Wright, a federal court of appeals judge, who issued the *ex parte* order. In his reasons, which he released five months later, he stated that "(t)he state as *parens patriae* will not allow a parent to abandon a child." Justice Wright also believed that the doctors and the hospital had a responsibility to treat Mrs Jones, and that, if they let her die, they were exposing themselves to civil and criminal liability.[252] He ignored the fact that both Mr and Mrs Jones had "volunteered to sign a waiver to relieve the hospital of any liability of the consequences of failure to effect the transfusion."[253]

While other trial followed suit and granted applications to permit the administration of blood transfusion on unwilling patients,[254] the *Georgetown* decision came under strong criticism.[255] Subsequent appellant courts who were called upon to consider the issue did not adopt the reasoning of Wright, which was found to be of "little precedential value"[256] and to have "extended the concept of abandonment ... into areas where it would conflict with other substantial interests."[257] Most appellant courts overturned orders violating the autonomous

---

[252] *Ibid.* Wright stated at p. 1009 "Mrs Jones was their responsibility to treat. The hospital doctors had the choice of administering the proper treatment or letting Mrs Jones die in the hospital bed, thus exposing themselves, and the hospital, to the risk of civil and criminal liability in either cases." A request for a rehearing en banc was denied. However, nine of the 10 federal judges who considered the Georgetown case would have denied the order.

[253] Baron, *Blood*, "Sin, and Death: Jehovah's Witnesses and the American Patients' Rights Movement," *supra* note 190, 108.

[254] See for example: *United States v. George*, 239 F. Supp. 752 (D. Conn. 1965); *Powell v. Columbian Presbyterian Medical Center*, 49 Mis. 2d 215, 267 N.Y.S.2d 450 (Sup. Ct. N.Y. County 1965); *In re Winthrop University Hospital*, 128 Misc. 2d 804, 490 N.Y.S.2d 996 (Sup. Ct. Nassau County 1985); *Crouse Irving Memorial Hospital, Inc. v. Paddock*, 127 Misc. 2d 101, 485 N.Y.S.2d 433 (Sup. Ct. Onondaga County 1985); *In re Jamaica Hospital*, 128 Misc. 2d 1006, 491 N.Y.S.2d 898 (Sup. Ct. Queens County 1985).

[255] Davis, "The Refusal of Life-Saving medical Treatment vs. the State's Interest in the Preservation of Life: A Clarification of the Interests at Stake," 85; Rhoden, "Litigating Life and Death," 381-2; Jonsen, "Blood Transfusions and Jehovah's Witnesses," 97-9; Note, "Compulsory Medical Treatment: The State's Interest Re-Evaluated," 292; Note, "The Refused Blood Transfusion: An Ultimate Challenge for Law and Morals," 202.

[256] *In re Dubreuil*, 629 So. 2d 819 at 824 n. 8.

[257] *Fosmire v. Nicoleau*, 551 N.E.2d 77 at 83.

right of competent adults to decide on medical treatment, even where third party interests were involved.[258] The common-law right to bodily integrity, the constitutional right to privacy, and the right to religious freedom, emerged as the foremost considerations when competing with third party interests.[259]

Another challenge to medical practitioners was the emergency scenario in which the now incompetent patient had either a relative available or advanced written directives, to establish that blood therapy was not consented to. Initially American courts held that "nothing less than a fully conscious, contemporaneous decision by the patient will be sufficient to override evidence of medical necessity."[260] However, in time, courts began to recognize a patient's "oral directives, actions or writings" as sufficient evidence to respect the refusal of a particular medical treatment deemed necessary by a physician.[261]

In Canada, where there was less litigation on the question of the right of medical decision making by a competent adult, the issue was thoroughly examined in 1990, by the Ontario Court of Appeal in the *Malette v. Shulman* case.[262] In this case, the treating physician administered a blood transfusion to an unconscious automobile accident victim who had in her wallet an *Advance*

---

[258] *In re Osborne*, 294 A.2d at 372 (D.C. 1972); *Public Health Trust v. Wons*, 541 So. 2d at 96 (Fla. 1989), 500 So. 2d at 679 (Fla. Dist. Ct. App. 1987); *Fosmire v. Nicoleau*, 75 N.Y.2d at 218, 551 N.E.2d at 77, 551 N.Y.S.2d at 876 (1990), 144 A.D.2d at 8, 536 N.Y.S.2d at 492 (1989); *Norwood Hospital v. Munoz*, 409 Mass. 116, 564 H.E.2d at 1017 (1991).

[259] See in general *In re Quinlan*, 70 N.J. 10, 355 A.2d 647 (1976) 617; *Superintendent of Belchertown State School v. Saikewicz*, Mass. 370 N.E. 2d 417 (1977); *In re Quackenbush*, 156 N.J. Super. 282, 383 A2d 785 (1978).

[260] *In re Estate of Dorone*, 502 A.2d 1271 (Pa. Super. 1985); See also *Werth v. Taylor*, 475 N.W.2d 426 (Mich. Ct. App. 1991).

[261] *In re Huges*, 259 N.J. Super. 193, 611 a.2d 1148 (App. Div. 1992).

[262] 67 D.L.R. (4th) 321 (Ont. C.A. 1990). On the matter of medical treatment for children, in *B. (R.) v. Children's Aid*, [1995] 1 S.C.R. 315, the Canadian Supreme Court decided that, while parents could not "refuse [for their children] medical treatment that is necessary and for which there is no reasonable alternative" (386), they did have the right to choose medical treatment for their children. "(T)he right to nurture a child, to care for its development, and to make decision for it in fundamental matters such as medical care, are part of the liberty interest of parents." (370) "the right of parents to rear their children according to their religious beliefs, including that of choosing medical and other treatments, is an equally fundamental aspect of freedom of religion."

Medical Directive indicating that she was one of Jehovah's Witnesses and did not consent to blood transfusion.[263] A few hours later, her daughter arrived at the hospital and confirmed to Dr Shulman that her mother did not want blood.[264] Dr Shulman refused to discontinue the transfusions. Mrs Malette eventually recovered and sued. The trial court ruled in favor of Mrs Malette. Dr Shulman was found guilty of battery and condemned to pay her $20,000 in damages.

The Ontario Court of Appeal, after considering the issues of the state's interest to preserve life,[265] the physician's dedication to saving lives, and the question of refusal for religious reasons, upheld the trial decision and, giving priority to self-determination, stated: "The right of a person to control his or her own body is a concept that has long been recognized at common law. The tort of battery has traditionally protected the interest in bodily security from unwanted physical interference. Basically, any intentional nonconsensual touching which is harmful or offensive to a person's reasonable sense of dignity is actionable."[266]

On the matter of refusing a medical treatment on religious grounds, the court wrote: "However sacred life may be, fair social comment admits that certain aspects of life are properly held to be more important than life itself. Such proud and honorable motivations are long entrenched in society, whether it be for patriotism in war, duty by law enforcement officers, protection of the life of a

---

263 See page 143 for a sample of the Advance Medical Directive carried by Mrs Malette.

264 *Ibid.*, 249. According to the daughter's evidence, Dr Shulman responded: "Don't you care if your mother dies? You will be responsible. I am in charge. I am responsible and I will give blood."

265 *Ibid.*, 336. On the matter of the state's interest, Justice Robins wrote: "The state's interest in persevering the life or health of a competent patient must generally give way to the patient's stronger interest in directing the course of her own life. As indicated earlier, there is no law prohibiting a patient from declining necessary treatment or prohibiting a doctor from honoring the patient's decision. To the extent that the law reflects the state's interest, it supports the right of individuals to make their own decisions. By imposing civil liability on those who perform medical treatment without consent even though the treatment may be beneficial, the law serves to maximize individual freedom of choice. Recognition of the right to reject medical treatment cannot, in my opinion, be said to depreciate the interest of the state in life or in the sanctity of life. Individual free choice and self-determination are themselves fundamental constituents of life. To deny individuals freedom of choice with respect to their health care can only lessen, and not enhance, the value of life."

266 *Malette v. Shulman, supra* note 269, 327.

spouse, son or daughter, death before dishonor, death before loss of liberty, or religious martyrdom. Refusal of medical treatment on religious grounds is such a value."[267]

Commenting on the validity of the *Advance Medical Directive* carried by Mrs Malette, the court concluded that it "set forth unqualified instructions applicable to the circumstances presented by this emergency. In the absence of any evidence to the contrary, those 'clear, precise and unequivocal' instructions should have been taken as validly representing the patient's wish not to be transfused."[268] The court understood and accepted that by carrying the *Advance Medical Directive* with her, Mrs Malette "gave notice to the doctor and the hospital, in the only practical way open to her, of her firm religious convictions as a Jehovah's Witness and her resolve to abstain from blood."[269]

Physicians in Canada have, for the most part, respected the *Malette* decision and have accepted to abide by the wishes of adult Jehovah's Witness patients as expressed by their *Advance Medical Directive*.[270]

A review of the case law involving Jehovah's Witness patients both in the United States and in Canada reveals a steady decline in cases being brought before

---

267 *Ibid.*, 272. See also comments by Adams, "Respecting the Right to Be Wrong," 753; Zeitz, "Legal Reasoning and Medical Decision Making," 755.

268 *Ibid.*, 337.

269 *Ibid.*, 335. Justice Robin of the Court of Appeal is here quoting the trial judge. The trial judge also added: "The card itself presents a clear, concise statement, essentially stating, "As a Jehovah's Witness, I refuse blood." That message is unqualified. It does not exempt life threatening perils. On the face of the card, its message is seen to be rooted in religious conviction." *Malette v. Shulman & al.*, 63 O.R. (2d) 243 at 268 (Ont. Sup. Ct., 1987).

270 See for example *Evelyn Estrella v. Princess Margaret Hospital & al.*, 2 June 1999, Court. File No. 99-CV-170514. This case involved a 39-year-old single woman suffering from leukemia. According to court documents, she had signed an *Advance Medical Directive* requesting that no blood be administered. The hospital chart also indicated that she had also verbally refused at least 15 times. Nevertheless, a nurse and a doctor were overheard badgering her to change her mind. Blood was eventually administered. As soon as the patient regained consciousness, she had her lawyer petition the court for an injunction restraining all hospital staff involved in her care "from communicating with the Plaintiff/Applicant Evelyn Estrella with respect to receiving blood transfusions, other than recommending such treatment" and prohibiting doctors "from administering blood transfusions" unless proper consent was obtained. The injunction was granted.

the courts. No doubt the involvement of the Hospital Liaison Committees[271] has played a significant role, as has the emergence of bloodless medicine following the blood scandals of the 1980s. Also, "because medicine is always practiced in a climate of uncertainty, where the facts are not and cannot be known, no analysis can produce the 'right' clinical decision."[272] Thus, it is not surprising that, in many cases where courts had been told by treating physician that the patient's life was threatened without the use of blood, the patient was successfully managed without blood.[273]

The right of a person to control his or her own body has also been extended to 'mature minors' by both courts and legislators.[274] For example, in the Province of Quebec, the *Civil Code* provides that if a minor is 14 years old or more, a doctor may not override a refusal for medical treatment unless a court order has

---

271 See *infra*, Chapter 1, section C, number 1: Hospital Liaison Committees.

272 Lehmann, "Decision Analysis: A Language for Survival in the Era of Managed Care," 69.

273 For example see: (This information as supplied by W. Glen How & Associates from the Watchtower Society Canada Branch) *In re Rena*, 705 N.E.2d 1155 (Mass. Ct. App. 1999) (medical evidence of the "potential need" of blood products, minor patient with lacerated spleen was managed without blood); *In re Harrell*, 678 So. 2d 455 (Fla. Dist. Ct. App. 1996) (in doctor's opinion pregnant patient had "a life-threatening blood condition" yet she received no blood); *In re W.M.*, 823 S.W. 2d 128 (Mo. Ct. App. 1992) (doctor testified that minor patient absolutely needed platelet and red cell transfusions yet patient was transferred to other facility and was successfully treated without blood); *McKenzie v. Doctors' Hosp. of Hollywood, Inc.*, 765 F. Supp. 1504, 1505 (S.D. Fla. 1991) (ex parte order obtained to administer to patient 'life-saving' transfusion but patient left before the transfusion was administered and was treated in another center without the use of blood); *Norwood Hosp. v. Munoz*, 564 N.E. 2d 1017, 1019-20 (Mass. 1991) (Doctor argued that blood was "reasonably necessary" yet patient was managed without blood); *Mercy Hosp., Inc. v. Jackson*, 489 A.2d 1130, 1131 (Md. Ct. Spec. App. 1985) (Caesarian section successfully performed without blood in spite of doctors claiming "high risk of mortality" and "fatal risk" if blood was not ordered); *Lakeshore General Hospital v. Methot-Gaudreault*, Sup. Ct. Montreal, no. 500-05-008750-844, 1 August 1984 (*ex parte* court order allowing blood to be administered to a 20-year-old woman suffering from *post partum* hemorrhage – before order was carried out, she transferred to nearby hospital and was treated without blood); *In re Osborne*, 294 A.2d 372, 376 n.6 (D.C. 1972) (doctors petitioned Court to obtain order to administer 'needed' transfusions for trauma injuries, the petition was denied and patient successfully treated without blood).

274 See for example: *Region 2 Hospital Corp. v. Walker*, 4 R.F.L. (4th) 321 (New Brunswick Ct. App. 1994) (15-year-old with acute myeloid leukemia); *Re A.Y.*, 111 348 A.P.R. 91 (Nfld. Fam. Ct. 1993) (15-year-old boy suffering from cancer; *Re L.D.K.*, 48 R.F.L. (2d) 164 (Ont. Prov. Ct.) (12-year-old girl suffering from leukemia); In British Colombia, *Infants Act*, *R.S.B.C.* 1979, c. 196 recognizes right of competent minor (no age limit) to consent to medical treatment; In New Brunswick, *Medical Consent of Minors Act*, N.B. Acts, 1979, c. 41 provides for two doctors to decide if minor under 16 has capacity to decide on treatment.

been obtained.[275]

Jehovah's Witnesses have not limited their effort to fighting court battles over the issue of the right of a patient to medical decision making. They have also embarked on an extensive campaign to support their members and educate health-care professionals.

[275] Article 14 of the *Quebec Civil Code* allows for "a minor fourteen years of age or over" to consent alone to medical care. Article 16 states that court authorization is necessary to force "a minor fourteen years of age or over to undergo care he refuses, except in the case of emergency if his life is in danger or his integrity threatened, in which case the consent of the person having parental authority or the tutor is sufficient." Cases in the province involving Jehovah's Witness minors over 14 years old have generally been dealt with by health care professionals, without going to court. Mr Alain Beauchemin, coordinator of the Montreal area Hospital Liaison Committee for Jehovah's Witnesses, submitted the following information in a personal interview: "Since the adoption of the new *Civil Code*, physicians have been respecting the wishes of mature minors over 14 years old. For example, a 16-year-old female was transferred from New Brunswick following a serious car accident where she suffered severe injuries to her intestines and spleen. She refused blood and her wishes were respected. In another case, a 16-year-old male requested no blood be administered during surgery. The anesthesiologist considered asking for a court order, but was counseled by the Hospital attorney to respect the wishes of the individual. No blood was administered. Finally, in another case, a 14-year-old male was admitted to the hospital with leukemia. Once it was determined that the young man was competent to decide on medical treatment, his wishes were respected. However, since the beginning of 2001 there has been a tendency by hospitals in Quebec and in different parts of Canada to petition the court when a minor refuses a blood transfusion. In one case from Alberta in 2002, a 16 and a half year-old girl suffering from acute myeloid leukemia refused blood transfusions. The court ordered the transfusions to be administered against her will. She was restrained, sedated and administered multiple transfusions. Eventually she died."

3. Effective Alternatives

Blood as the 'gift of life' continues to be a strongly entrenched perception. Not surprisingly, Jehovah's Witnesses, in objecting to this 'queen of remedies,' have sometimes been perceived as religious zealots seeking martyrdom, or even as "medical nihilists."[276] Adjudicators, social workers and the public in general have at times judged their position as unreasonable, irrational and irresponsible. Often passing unnoticed in the debate is that blood therapy is the only treatment that Jehovah's Witnesses, as a group, refuse. And furthermore, there are now numerous effective alternatives to blood transfusion.[277] According to one prominent physician, the Witnesses readily seek out "the best in medical treatment" and as a group are "among the most educated consumers the surgeon will ever encounter."[278]

As discussed earlier, Jehovah's Witnesses believe their refusal of blood transfusion to be an important fundamental Biblical teaching. They are not concerned that mainstream Christian religions disagree with them on this doctrine.[279] Some of this disagreement may be due to a lack of accurate

---

[276] Nielsen, "The Biblical Laws Against Transfusions Reexamined – A Christian Physician's Viewpoint," 273. This author sees in the refusal of blood transfusion for religious reasons "a smattering of martyrdom.;" Spence, Clinical Practice of Transfusion Medicine, *infra* note 372, 600.

[277] See *infra* Chapter 1, section C, number 3: Medical Alternatives to Blood Transfusion.

[278] Spence, Clinical Practice of Transfusion Medicine, *infra* note 372 of chapter 4, 602.

[279] Boyd, Critical Care – Standards, Audit and Ethics, 393. In this article, the author states that "no major religion for which the Biblical scriptures are authoritative endorses the Jehovah's Witnesses' interpretation of the texts on which their opposition to blood transfusion is based." This leads him to ask: "In the light of the religious consensus that Jehovah's Witnesses are mistaken in their interpretation of Scripture … Why is this particular religious belief, so clearly rejected by other religious authorities, now so clearly defended in law as to discharge doctors of their normal responsibilities …?" It would seem that to analyze the beliefs of a minority religious group in light of mainstream religions and to conclude that, since the majority does not agree, the group in question must be mistaken, is to endorse what the Canadian Supreme Court called the "tyranny of the majority." See *Chaput v. Romain*

information regarding their refusal[280] or may simply be theological dispute.[281]

Furthermore, Witnesses are convinced that God's command to abstain from blood is not only for their future eternal welfare, but also for their immediate temporal benefit. They maintain their stand is a reasonable one "vindicated by a flood of new scientific findings on both the dangers of homologous transfusions and the safety of alternatives to transfusion."[282] In their view, obeying God on this issue has shown that non-blood medical management can be more beneficial

---

& al., [1955] S.C.R. 834.

280 See for example Verhey, Religious Methods and Resources in Bioethics, 263. Verhey is of the view that Jehovah's Witnesses have a "curious reading of a curious set of texts about blood" which is in fact an 'abuse of scripture' which has harmed "marginalized patients," "usually women and children." This view seems to be contradicted by physicians who have observed first hand that Witness patients "think deeply and pray earnestly about decisions regarding blood transfusions," seek the "best in medical treatment, ... are among the most educated consumers" and have 'done better' when undergoing major surgery such as open-heart surgery without the use of blood. Spence, Clinical Practice of Transfusion Medicine, *infra* note 372 of chapter 4, 602; Adams, "Respecting the Right to Be Wrong," *supra* note 267 (of chapter 2), 753; Kay, "Need for Blood in Open-Heart Surgery," 1230.

281 See Muramoto, "Bioethics of the Refusal of Blood by Jehovah's Witnesses: Part 1. Should Bioethical Deliberation Consider Dissident's Views?" 230; Muramoto, "Bioethics of the Refusal of Blood by Jehovah's Witnesses: Part 2. A Novel Approach Based on Rational Non-Interventional Paternalism," 301. In these articles, Dr Muramoto advocates leaving the medical arena to engage in a theological "in-depth discussion" on the doctrine of blood with patients who are Jehovah's Witnesses. The purpose of the interchange would be to convince them that their understanding of the scriptures is wrong. He has also set up a website which appears to rely heavily on material from disgruntled ex-members of Jehovah's Witnesses. D. Malyon, Chairman of the Hospital Liaison Committee of Jehovah's Witnesses in Luton, England responded to Muramoto articles which he "consider(ed) outside and unwelcome to ethical debate." He quoted an Italian sociologist and international expert in new religious movements. This expert expresses concern regarding the "unreliability and the unrepresentative nature of the views of former members of religious organizations." Malyon attributes Muramoto's apparent hostility to Jehovah's Witnesses to personal motives: "At least he (Muramoto) has the honesty to declare his motives on his public website on the Internet, where he openly admits to religious differences with his own Jehovah's Witness wife." See Malyon, "Transfusion-Free Treatment of Jehovah's Witnesses: Respecting the Autonomous Patient's Rights," 302, 376; See also Green, "Biblical Laws Relating to Blood Transfusion: The Judaic Laws and Principles," 247.

282 "Bridging the Gap Between Doctors and Witness Patients," Awake!, 21. On the risks associated with blood transfusion see: Dobroszcki, "A Cluster of Transfusion-Associated Babesiosis Cases Traced to a Single Asymptomatic Donor," 927; Sazama, "Adverse Effects of Blood Transfusion," 451; Saéz-Alquézar, "Evaluation of the Performance of Brazilian Blood Banks in Testing for Chagas' Disease," 228; Williamson, "Reporting Serious Hazards of Transfusion: The SHOT Program," 28; Grzelak, "Blood Transfusions Downregulate Hematopoiesis and Subsequently Downregulate the Immune Response," 1104; Wolf & Gold, Blood Conservation in Cardiac Surgery 7; Fakhry, Textbook of Surgery 118, 124-5; Blumberg, "Allogenic Transfusion and Infection: Economic and Clinical Implications," 34; Tartter, "Immunologic Effects of Blood Transfusions," 277; Krever, "Interim Report" Commission of Inquiry on the Blood System in Canada, *supra* note 3, 17-33.

and less dangerous than blood therapy.[283]

To counter public misconception and to provide assistance and support for members whose treating physician deems blood is necessary in their situation, Jehovah's Witnesses have launched a research and education campaign that includes the following:

- Establishment of Hospital Liaison Committees in larger cities worldwide.
- Extensive research of medical literature on alternatives to blood and blood products.
- Direct contact with health-care professionals to inform them about the position of Jehovah's Witnesses and to discuss available alternative treatments.

Hospital Liaison Committees

In the early 1960s, the headquarters of Jehovah's Witnesses started compiling a list of cooperative physicians familiar with medical alternatives to blood transfusion. This information was shared with local congregations as the need arose.[284] Eventually, the need for better communication between the Witnesses and the medical community led to the establishment of Hospital Liaison Committees. The initial project was piloted by their Canadian Branch and

283 "The Most Precious Fluid in the World," Awake!, 15: "Furthermore, abstaining from blood transfusions has protected Witnesses from myriads of dangers. More and more people besides Jehovah's Witnesses are refusing blood transfusions today. Slowly the medical community is responding and reducing its use of blood. As the Surgery Annual put it: "Clearly, the safest transfusion is the one not given." Witnesses have also printed accounts of individuals who escaped the ravages of the blood scandals because they refused blood products. See "My Life With Hemophilia," Awake!, 21. (Account John A. Wortendyke, who suffered from severe hemophilia and upon becoming one of Jehovah's Witnesses in 1972 ceased to take blood products. His condition was managed without blood and he was still alive in 1987.) "Canada's 'Tainted Blood' Inquiry," Awake!, 22. (Account of William Hall, a 76-year-old Jehovah's Witness man, with severe hemophilia, who testified before the Canadian Krever Commission on tainted blood about how "he successfully manages his condition using alternatives to blood products." Mr Hall testified that his bother also had hemophilia: "He didn't have the same faith [religion] as I have, so he took a blood transfusion and he died from hepatitis.")

284 "Doctor-Patient Communication – A Key to Success," Awake!, 12.

was so successful that it eventually developed into a worldwide network. From a handful in 1979, the number of Hospital Liaison Committees has grown to over 1,200 in 200 countries. They describe themselves as "an international network of experienced ministers who are trained to liaise with medical personnel at the patient's request." Support is given to members as well as to treating physicians by "arranging consults with doctors and medical teams experienced in bloodless medicine and surgery techniques."[285]

These committees operate under the direction of the Watch Tower Society Hospital Information Services (HIS) located at their international headquarters in Brooklyn as well as in major branches around the world.[286] Members of the Hospital Liaison Committees are chosen from among experienced local ministers and receive extensive ongoing training to help qualify them to work with doctors, social workers, judges and hospital personnel. They provide the following

---

[285] Hospital Liaison Committee for Jehovah's Witnesses, form HIS-1 11/96.

[286] Mr Zenon Bodnaruk, Director of Hospital Information Services (HIS) for Canada supplied the following information regarding the services offered by HIS:

"Hospital Information Services (Canada) is part of an international network disseminating authoritative information regarding strategies to avoid allogeneic blood transfusion and facilitating access to health care for patients who are Jehovah's Witnesses.

HIS facilitates, at no cost to the physician, access to current and clinically relevant information regarding strategies to avoid allogeneic blood transfusion. Our services to physicians include the following:

- Ongoing searches of the leading peer-reviewed medical journal for advances in blood conservation and management of patients without transfusion and periodic mailings of clinically useful information.
- Literature search service for specific clinical questions regarding blood management options for patients who are Jehovah's Witnesses.
- Concise summaries and bibliographies of nonblood management strategies.
- Speakers arranged for grand rounds, seminars, etc., on medical and ethical issues in the care of Witness patients.
- Support to physicians and Witness patients through local representatives of the Hospital Liaison Committee Network.
- Facilitate consults with medical specialists (in Canada and the US) with special expertise in the use of medical alternatives to allogeneic transfusion.
- Contacts with hospitals (now 200 in 20 countries) with formalized blood conservation or "bloodless" medicine and surgery programs."

services:

- Facilitate consults with over 30,000 doctors in Canada and the U.S., over 100,000 worldwide.
- International contacts with bloodless medicine and surgery programs.
- Arrange patient transfers.
- A specialized information service for doctors and access to over 4,000 medical and scientific publications for on-line medical researchers.
- Presentations to medical staff.
- Expertise on informed consent policy development.
- Consultation on bloodless medicine and surgery programs.
- Assistance in cases where court orders are sought.[287]

In every city where they are located they have established an emergency phone number where they can be reached by local congregations, hospitals or treating physicians. A 24-hour National Hot Line has been set up in most countries. The Witness periodical *Awake!* keeps members abreast of progress made by Hospital Liaison Committees throughout the world as well as their efforts to contact favorable doctors and assist members who need medical alternatives to homologous blood.[288] They have supplied information to physicians that "disabuses them of mistaken notions regarding the necessity of

---

[287] *Ibid.*

[288] "Bridging the Gap Between Doctors and Witness Patients," Awake!, 21. (Reports from Australia, New Zealand, Philippines, Hong Kong , Taiwan, Japan and Korea.); "Doctor-Patient Communication – A Key to Success," Awake!, 12. (Accounts of individual members being helped by the Hospital Liaison Committees); "Pioneering Bloodless Surgery with Jehovah's Witnesses," Awake!, 8. (Reports from England, Sweden, France, Germany, Spain, Mexico, Brazil, Puerto Rico and U.S.A.); "Jehovah's Witnesses and the Medical Profession Cooperate," Awake!, 24 (Reports from Australia, France and U.S.A.); "Seminars to Improve Relations Between Doctors and Jehovah's Witnesses," Awake!, 19 (Letter from Doctor Pope who attended a seminar put on by Hospital Liaison Committee in the San Francisco Bay area.).

transfusions and makes them aware of neglected techniques for treating patients without blood."[289] Through the information provided by the Hospital Liaison Committees, Jehovah's Witnesses have become more knowledgeable on medical issues that concern them.[290]

Articles in medical journals, as well as in their own publications, indicate that Jehovah's Witnesses have gone to great lengths to support members who refuse blood therapy. In fact, it is doubtful that any other international consortium is as vast or as efficient, specializing in the gathering and distribution of medical research on one particular topic, in this case – medical alternatives to blood transfusion.

Educational campaign

In recent years, Hospital Liaison Committees in various parts of the world have been involved in seminars for health-care professionals where the benefits of bloodless medicine are discussed. In 1998, *Awake!* reported four such seminars involving more than 1,400 professionals from 12 countries.[291] During the 25th Congress of the International Society of Blood Transfusion, held in Oslo, Norway, in 1998 and attended by over 1,700 doctors from 83 countries, Hospital Information Services set up an exhibition booth where doctors could obtain handouts containing abstracts of some 1,000 medical articles. Information on medical techniques that eliminate the need for blood transfusions during surgery was also available.[292]

In 1982, Jehovah's Witnesses in France set up an association called *Association médico-scientifique d'information et d'assistance du malade* (AMS)

---

[289] Baron, Blood, Sin, and Death: Jehovah's Witnesses and the American Patients' Rights Movement, *supra* note 190 of chapter 2, 9.

[290] Spence, Clinical Practice of Transfusion Medicine, *infra* note 372 of chapter 4, 602.

[291] "Doctors Take a New Look at Bloodless Surgery," Awake!, 18.

[292] "Nonblood Treatment – What Experts Say," Awake!, 19.

which involves both Witness and non-Witness professionals. Through this association, they have organized "several national and regional meetings and lent support to work on research, theses, and medical liability articles."[293] Members from this association have participated in medical conferences in different parts of Europe, Eastern Europe and Africa, promoting bloodless medicine.

The *Canadian Medical Association Journal* reported in 1996 on efforts by the Hospital Information Services to "educate the medical community about the Jehovah's Witnesses position on blood and to promote 'bloodless' medicine and surgery in Canada." According to this report, representatives had visited more than 10 medical schools and 200 hospitals across the country. Some universities include a presentation from Hospital Information Services as part of an undergraduate curriculum unit. The presentation includes a brief overview of medical treatment Jehovah's Witnesses accept and that they object to, an explanation of their religious beliefs, a discussion of the ethical and legal issues involved, and an explanation of how Hospital Information Services (HIS) through access to experienced specialists, Hospital Liaison Committees (HLC), and online research, can assist doctors treating church members.[294]

According to church officials, many students and doctors who attended

---

[293] A.M.S., Le refus des transfusions sanguines, 6. See also: 'Compte rendu du colloque de Bordeaux du 8 novembre 1986"l'Association médico-scientifique d'information et d'assistance du malade (Montfort Lamaury, 1986). Following this conference, AMS published a 32-page brochure entitled *Sauver des vies sans violer des consciences*, addressed to healthcare professionals; Another seminar was organized in 1993 entitled *Les Témoins de Jéhovah, le droit de la famille, de la santé, du service national et les libertés publiques*, at which American professor Charles Baron was invited to present his paper *Blood, Sin, and Death: Jehovah's Witnesses and the American patient Rights Movement*, which he had already presented earlier that year at a seminar held at the University of Paris X (Nanterre). Another seminar entitled *Ateliers épargne sanguine*, held on 27 January 1994 at which a handout (not published) containing 17 abstracts of presentations by doctors and professors on bloodless medicine was circulated. At the 10th World Congress on Medical Law, held in Jerusalem, in 1994, Philippe Goni, attorney for Jehovah's Witnesses and associated with A.M.S. presented a paper entitled *"Aspects juridiques du refus d'un malade de se soumettre à un traitment médical"*; For an example of some of their articles, see: Garay & Goni, "La valeur juridique de l'attestation de refus de transfusion sanguine," 14; Delmas & Garay, "Le Bureau d'information hospitalier des Témoins de Jéhovah," 36-8; Najand, "Anesthésiste-réanimateur et Témoins de Jéhovah," 237.

[294] Robb, "Jehovah's Witnesses Leading Education Drive as Hospitals Adjust to No Blood Requests," 557.

these presentations expressed amazement at the large number of available alternatives to transfusion. They were also surprised by the extent of the support network for physicians and patients as well as the information services provided to physicians by HIS and HLCs.[295]

Within this education campaign, the Watch Tower Society has published a volume entitled *Family Care and Medical Management for Jehovah's Witnesses* which has been distributed to many professionals involved in health-care decisions involving church members, including physicians, judges and social workers. This reference manual can be found in most hospital libraries. It contains information about the Worldwide Hospital Liaison Committee Network (1,200 committees servicing 200 countries), phone numbers to contact local committees, suggested hospital protocol for treating Jehovah's Witnesses,[296] a review of their beliefs, ethical, legal and social factors to consider, as well as information on extensive medical research into bloodless medicine. It is published in a three-ring binder format and is updated regularly.

Medical alternatives to blood transfusion

While surgeons have been taught since the 1920s the 'halstedian principles' of minimizing blood loss during surgery,[297] the popularity of 'bloodless medicine'

---

[295] This information was supplied by Mr Zenon Bodnaruk, Director of Hospital Information Services (Canada) for Jehovah's Witnesses in an interview on 23 July 1999.

[296] The protocol suggested is the following: "PURSUE nonblood medical alternatives, and treat the patient without using homologous blood; CONSULT with other doctors experienced in non blood medical management at the same facility, and treat without using homologous blood; CONTACT local Hospital Liaison Committee of Jehovah's Witnesses to locate cooperative doctors at other facilities for consultation on alternative medical care; TRANSFER patient, if necessary, to cooperative doctor or facility before patient's condition deteriorates; IN A RARE SITUATION, if the above steps have been exhausted and governmental intervention is deemed necessary, the patient, the parents, or the guardian should be notified as soon as possible of such intended action." Family Care and Medical Management for Jehovah's Witnesses, EMERGENCY 5.

[297] William Steward Halsted advocated in the 1920s "careful diagnosis and planning before surgery, gentle tissue handling, incisions along avascular anatomic planes to avoid vessels, and meticulous hemostasis." He stressed the importance of preventing blood loss over replacing blood loss. See Halsted, Surgical Papers.

is a relatively new phenomenon, resulting largely from the widely publicized tainted blood scandals. Jehovah's Witnesses, though, have been advocating bloodless medicine for years.

Since Jehovah's Witnesses object to being administered blood, not to medical treatment in general, it is understandable that they would champion the cause for bloodless medicine. To facilitate their access to good healthcare they have sought to establish that: 1) their objection is reasonable, rational, and supported by medical literature; 2) alternatives to blood and blood products are safer, therefore obeying God's law has immediate benefits.

While there still exists much 'confusion, emotional bias, intolerance and ignorance' among doctors regarding the treatment of Jehovah's Witnesses, this is not the case with all health-care professionals. A growing number from the medical community have tried to promote the development "of a positive philosophy towards" Witnesses by advocating careful preoperative and intra-operative management, as well as the use of specialized anesthetic techniques.[298]

As early as 1964, open heart operations were successfully performed on Witnesses without the use of blood. In 1974, Dr D. Cooley wrote: "Encouraging results in our group of Jehovah's Witness patients support our belief that the commitment not to transfuse blood is not an obstacle to the successful performance of such major surgery as aorto-coronary bypass with the saphenous vein."[299] In another case, following some 6,000 open-heart operations at St.Vincent's Hospital, in Los Angeles, during which most of the patients did not receive blood, it was a doctor's "impression that the patients do better" without

---

298 Minuck & Lambie, "Anesthesia and Surgery for Jehovah's Witnesses," *infra* note 373 of chapter 5. See also Malyon, "Transfusion-Free Treatment of Jehovah's Witnesses: Respecting the Autonomous Patient's Motives," *supra* note 281, 381. Malyon, who is Chairman of Hospital Liaison Committee of Jehovah's Witnesses in Luton, England writes: "The atmosphere between members of our faith and the medical profession as a whole is becoming increasingly relaxed and even friendly."

299 Sandiford, "Aorta-Coronary Bypass in Jehovah's Witnesses," 1.

the use of blood.[300] Other doctors began noticing these impressive results. In 1978, Dr Englbert Dunfhy wrote: "We have had a number of patients at our hospital over the last 12 years who have been Jehovah's Witnesses, and we have operated without blood transfusions. I may be wrong, but I cannot recall a patient who died because of lack of transfusion. ... Transfusion certainly makes the surgeon feel better, but it may not make the patient feel better. Perhaps we all have a tendency to transfuse to make ourselves more comfortable. I think when we have a Jehovah's Witness, we'll do well to consider his point of view."[301]

The development of bloodless medicine in the 1970s and 1980s was mainly due to favorable physicians who were willing to treat Jehovah's Witnesses while respecting their conscientious objection to blood.[302] This happened at a time when blood products, still considered the 'queen of remedies' continued to be

---

[300] Kay, "Need for Blood in Open-Heart Surgery," *supra* note 280, 1230.

[301] In the *Bulletin* of the American College of Surgeons, June, 1978, Dr Englbert Dunphy, from San Francisco, made the following comments: "(Lord) Hunt goes on to make a final plea for better training of medical students, doctors, and clergy in the meanings of religion in different areas. Hunt made his plea ten years ago, and we are just beginning to heed it now in this country. We know the problems associated with Jehovah's Witnesses. We have had a number of patients at our hospital over he last 12 years who have been Jehovah's Witnesses, and we have operated without blood transfusions. I may be wrong, but I cannot recall a patient who died because of lack of transfusion. I agree, however, a patient may have become anemic through the course of the day."

"I was fascinated to find a paper just published by Denton Cooley reporting on more than 500 major cardiac operations involving Jehovah's Witnesses performed without transfusion and showing a mortality rate of 5 percent. The figures are comparable to his figures on patients given adequate transfusion."

"Transfusion certainly makes the surgeon feel better, but it may not make the patient feel better. Perhaps we all have a tendency to transfuse to make ourselves more comfortable. I think when we have a Jehovah's Witness, we'll do well to consider his point of view."

[302] Kambouris, "Major Abdominal Operations on Jehovah's Witnesses," 350. (Thirteen major operations successfully performed on 11 Jehovah's Witness patients without complications.) Garcia, "Anemia and Anesthesia," 15. (Surgery and general anesthesia on over 10,000 Jehovah's Witness patients without the use of blood or blood products.) "Two Hospitals Offering Patients Options of "Bloodless Surgery," 50. (Bloodless surgery program offered to all patients of the Graduate Hospital in Philadelphia. Over 5,000 operations performed without transfusions on both Witnesses and non-Witnesses at Pioneer Park Medical Center, in Texas.) Bonakdar, "Major Gynecologic and Obstetric Surgery on Jehovah's Witnesses," 587. (Retrospective study of 165 Jehovah's Witnesses and 164 control patients showed no deaths and few complications in both groups.) Nelson, "Total Hip Arthroplasty in Jehovah's Witnesses without Blood Transfusion," 350. (One hundred patients who were Jehovah's Witnesses successfully underwent total hip replacement without blood transfusion.)

used indiscriminately by medical professionals.

However, by the end of the 1980s, the medical community was "jolted into awareness of the risks involved in blood transfusions by the (then) recent evidence linking transfusion with transmission of" AIDS.[303] Some believe that AIDS, at least partly, is a "consequence of the dramatic growth of blood transfusion networks in post World War II industrial societies."[304] At any rate, it became apparent that there were major problems with the blood supply. In 1993, Mark Boyd, director of gynecology at the Royal Victoria Hospital, in Montreal, noted: "Blood is not a popular product these days. Patients are frightened."[305] One of the recommendations of the Canadian Krever Commission,[306] in its 1995 interim report, was to inform patients "well in advance" to "enable them to employ some of the alternatives to an allogeneic blood transfusion."[307] Through the media, the public became educated about the risks associated with blood products and learned of available alternatives.[308] As a result, more patients were asking for alternatives to blood transfusion. In fact, there are reports that some patients would even falsely claim to be Jehovah's Witnesses so they could get a non-blood alternative to a blood transfusion.[309] A 1996 Gallup poll indicated that as many as 89% of Canadians, "if informed they required a blood transfusion due to a

---

303 Spence, "The Effects of Hemoglobin Levels and Blood Loss on Surgical Mortality," 264. See also Spence, "Elective Surgery without Transfusion: Influence of Preoperative Hemoglobin Level and Blood Loss on Mortality," 320.

304 Wailoo, Drawing Blood, 13.

305 Rafuse, "Better Planning Could Have Saved Life of Woman Who Refused Transfusion, MD says," 1596. See also Polk, "Blood Management Practice Guidelines: Conference Highlights," 15: "the public's awareness of new pathogens has made blood transfusion a less attractive treatment option."

306 Mr Justice Krever was appointed Commissioner by the Canadian government in 1993 to inquire into and report on the blood system in Canada. See Interim Report, Commission of Inquiry of the Blood System in Canada.

307 *Ibid.*, 66.

308 See for example Jenish, "Bad Blood," 22; "Le sang," 494; Picard, "Tragedy Prompts Bloodless Solutions," A1, A8; Bueckert, "Bloodless Medicine Continuing to Gain in Popularity," A10.

309 Bragg, "Fake Witnesses Avoid Transfusions," A9.

surgical operation," would chose an alternative to donor blood.[310] In England, 'hemovigilance' led to the setting up of the SHOT (Serious Hazards of Transfusion) program intended "to receive and collate confidential reports of transfusion fatalities and major complications."[311]

Blood conservation policies were put in place in most hospitals resulting in a decrease of the number of patients being transfused.[312] Blood conservation programs include preoperative patient preparation (treatment of anemia and/or clotting deficiencies, and minimal phlebotomy for lab testing). Surgical techniques include the use of hemostatic scalpels, minimally invasive procedures and surgical techniques designed to minimize blood loss, and for emergency situations: prompt arrest of bleeding, hemostatic agents, and appropriate fluid management.[313] Physicians also developed techniques such as controlled hypotension, hemodilution, intra- and postoperative blood salvage and reinfusion.[314] For example, up until 1985 there was no blood conservation program at the Ottawa Heart Institute and this resulted in 94% of their patients receiving transfused blood. However, after the adoption of a blood conservation

---

310 Quoted in Thomas, "Nonblood Management in Obstetrics and Gynecology," 475.

311 Williamson, "Reporting Serious Hazards of Transfusion: The SHOT Program," *supra* note 282, 28.

312 An example of an attempt by the medical profession to address its problem of blood management and conservation is seen in the "Blood Management Practice Guidelines Conference" held 12-14 January 1995 in Dallas, Texas. For full report on conference and papers presented see "Consensus Conference: Blood Management – Surgical Practice Guidelines," 1S.

313 Robblee, "Alternatives to Blood Transfusion: The Surgical Perspective" (Report of proceedings and recommendations of conference Building a Blood System the 21st Century, Toronto, 3-4 November 1997) 17. "In a series of 56 patients undergoing minimally invasive coronary bypass surgery at the Ottawa Heart Institute, only 1 patient (1.8%) needed a blood transfusion during surgery and this was a person with hemophilia." It is interesting to note the Denton Cooley had been using blood conservation methods since 1962 with good success on Jehovah's Witness patients. See Cooley., "Open Heart Surgery in Jehovah's Witnesses," 779; See also Spence, Clinical Practice of Transfusion Medicine, 521.

314 Robblee, "Alternatives to Blood Transfusion: The Surgical Perspective," *supra* note 313, 16-17. See also Sher, "The Blood Conservation Program at The Toronto Hospital" (Report of proceedings and recommendations of conference for *Building a Blood System the 21st Century*, Toronto, 3-4 November 1997) 46-8. See also Joseph, Blood Conservation in the Surgical Patient, 252. For early comments on the acceptability for Witnesses to accept blood salvage methods see "Questions from Readers," The

policy, the number of patients being administered blood transfusions decreased to 36% with no adverse effect on patient care.[315] The obvious benefit of this new program was that a large number of patients were not exposed to the risks associated with blood transfusions. The benefits of a restrictive transfusion strategy and avoidance of an arbitrary transfusion trigger have been confirmed by a recent Canadian clinical trial involving 838 patients. During the trial, it was found that in one particular group, when blood was used liberally, "one additional death occurred for every 13 patients." Significantly, the trial also revealed that when a restrictive strategy regarding the use of blood was adopted, the number of transfusions decreased by 54%.[316]

Another phenomenon of this new awareness to the dangers associated with blood transfusion therapy is the appearance of centers for bloodless medicine. In the United States the first center for bloodless medicine was established in 1987 at the Our Lady of Resurrection Medical Center in Chicago. While treating over 200 patients a year in their bloodless program, they observed that "(t)here is very little that can't be done" without blood, and patients who do not receive blood transfusion remain hospitalized "one day less on average compared with other patients with the same diagnosis."[317] David Rosencrantz, director of a bloodless center in Portland, stated that after treating 500 to 700 patients annually over a period of four years, he hadn't lost a single patient. He also found the program cost effective since these patients were out a full day earlier.[318]

Watchtower (15 October 1959), 640.

[315] Robblee, "Alternatives to Blood Transfusion: The Surgical Perspective," *supra* note 314, 16.

[316] Ely, "Transfusions in Critically Ill Patients," 468. See also, Hébert, "A Multicenter, Randomized, Controlled Clinical Trial of Transfusion Requirements in Critical Care," 409.

[317] Robb, "Jehovah's Witnesses Leading Education Drive as Hospitals Adjust to No Blood Requests," *supra* note 294, 559. See also deCastro, "Bloodless Surgery: Establishment of a Program for the Special Medical Needs of the Jehovah's Witness Community—The Gynecologic Surgery Experience at a Community Hospital," 1491. Bloodless program indicated high level of patient satisfaction and potential for improved patient care with no increase of morbidity.

[318] Robb, "Jehovah's Witnesses Leading Education Drive as Hospitals Adjust to No Blood Requests," *supra* note 294, 560.

By early 1996, there were more than 100 bloodless centers in the world, 52 of them in the U.S.A.[319] In 1999, the number in the U.S.A. had risen to 75 centers.[320]

According to David Davis, Associate Dean of Continuing Education at the University of Toronto's Faculty of Medicine, "a myth in the medical field is that when you research something and you publish it, or speak to a large conference, your colleagues will automatically change." The impetus must come from patients, and in the field of bloodless surgery, patients who are Jehovah's Witnesses are providing such an impetus.[321] As the momentum in the demand for bloodless medicine increased, the medical profession began taking note of the extensive research that had been gathered by Witnesses in their bid to educate health-care professionals on non-blood alternatives to blood transfusion therapy. In the "first ever multi-disciplinary conference of its kind in Canada, perhaps in the world," entitled *Building a Blood System for the 21st Century*, Witnesses were invited to participate in and to submit for publication, along with the report of the conference, a comprehensive 28-page paper on *Medical Alternatives to Blood Transfusions*.[322]

---

319 Picard, "Tragedy Prompts Bloodless Solutions," *supra* note 192, A8.

320 Dougherty, "La fin des transfusions?" L'Actualité, 18.

321 Picard, "Tragedy Prompts Bloodless Solutions," *supra* note 192 of chapter 2, A8.

322 "Medical Alternatives to Blood Transfusions" (Report of proceedings and recommendations of the conference *Building a Blood System the 21st Century*, Toronto, 3-4 November 1997) (1997) Hospital Information Services (Canada) for Jehovah's Witnesses 57-88.

4. A Profound Religious Belief

When considering a religiously based objection to a medical treatment, the role religion plays in the patient's life must be examined. The patient may have adopted a religion that encompasses a profound commitment to a certain lifestyle such as that of Jehovah's Witnesses.[323] To impose upon these patients medical treatment that violates their religiously trained conscience would be a gross violation of their human dignity and could have devastating moral and spiritual consequences.

Consideration for human dignity, as well as respect for a patient's values and preferences, imposes upon the physician a moral (and legal) obligation to treat the individual according to expressed wishes. In order to do this it is essential for the doctor to know and understand the patient, including any firmly held religious convictions. In the case of Jehovah's Witnesses this might include considering the following information.

The religion of Jehovah's Witnesses

Contrary to the assertion of some authors that this religious group is "very secretive" about its beliefs, Jehovah's Witnesses appear very unsecretive about their beliefs and values.[324] All of their religious meetings and conventions are

---

[323] The Supreme Court of Canadahas recognized that those who adopt such a religious lifestyle will often be "vulnerable to stereotype, social prejudice and marginalization." See *Adler v. Ontario,* [1996] 3 S.C.R. 607 at 661.

[324] For example, in Blajchman, "Transfusion-Related Issues in Jehovah's Witness Patients," 243 the author writes: "It has been quite difficult to determine just what the Witnesses' beliefs are, because they are very secretive about them." This statement is surprising considering the wide distribution of their literature. *The Watchtower*, Witnesses' main periodical contains an ongoing discussion of their

open to the general public.[325] In their 'trademark' door-to-door preaching activity, they freely discuss various religious and social topics with anyone who will listen.[326] Their publications, including the periodicals *THE WATCHTOWER* and *AWAKE!*, examine their religious beliefs and doctrines in detail and are widely circulated worldwide.[327] Apart from the Bible, *THE WATCHTOWER* is the main reference on doctrinal issues for Witnesses.[328] Information regarding their beliefs as well as their organizational structure is available to whoever may request it.

Why witnesses are so dedicated to their religion

Some doctors may express concern that the refusal to accept blood, rather than being motivated by personal conviction, may actually be an expression of blind adherence to a Church teaching of which the individual has little personal understanding. An appreciation of the process involved in becoming one of Jehovah's Witnesses may be useful in addressing this fear. Although prospective new Witnesses are regularly found by means of evangelizing activity, the conversion process is not a rapid one, nor is it based on an emotional experience.

The person interested in becoming one of Jehovah's Witnesses must first follow a structured and extensive Bible study course given on a one-to-one basis by a qualified congregation member. This in depth analysis of Bible and Church doctrine gives the student the opportunity to examine the reasons behind the teachings with a view to understanding them. Eventually, students are also expected to attend several weekly congregation meetings at the local church

---

beliefs and has an average printing of 22,328,000 copies every two weeks and is distributed publicly and from door-to-door worldwide in 131 languages. See The Watchtower (15 July 1999) 2.

325 Organized to Accomplish Our Ministry, 68.

326 Organized to Accomplish Our Ministry, *supra* note 325, 84.

327 These include such publications as Knowledge That Leads to Everlasting Life and You Can Live Forever in Paradise on Earth which contain a detailed discussion of their beliefs.

328 Organized to Accomplish Our Ministry, *supra* note 326, fr. 65.

(called *Kingdom Hall*) for further Bible study and to meet the requirements for sharing in the door to door preaching work.

This is a lifestyle religion that calls for commitment. For many candidates the process to conversion will require profound changes in their lives. Smoking, the use of recreational drugs, alcohol abuse, promiscuity, adultery and a host of other 'illicit' activities are not permitted. Since this moral code, believed to be Bible decreed, is strictly enforced, only very decided individuals convinced of the value of their newfound beliefs actually reach the point of qualifying for baptism. Before baptism, elders of the Church thoroughly review with the individual basic Bible doctrines, including the issue of blood transfusion as developed and explained in their literature, to ascertain that these have been well understood and accepted.[329] The individual must also personally and privately make a "dedication of his life to God," Only after all these steps, and if the person has clearly expressed "a sincere desire to obey its teachings (the Bible's) in harmony with Jehovah's Witnesses," is baptism possible.[330]

---

[329] The current Bible study aid used is Knowledge That Leads to Everlasting Life, *supra* note 327. On page 129, par. 22, the issue of blood is discussed:

"Jehovah told Noah and his family that blood represents the soul, or life. Therefore, God forbade them to eat any blood. (Genesis 9:3,4) Since we are their descendants, that law is binding upon all of us. Jehovah told the Israelites that blood was to be poured out on the ground and was not to be used for man's own purposes. (Deuteronomy 12:15, 16) And God's law on blood was reiterated when first-century Christians were instructed: "Keep abstaining...from blood." (Acts 15:28, 29) Out of respect for the sanctity of life, godly people do not accept blood transfusions, even if others insist that such a procedure would be lifesaving. Many medical alternatives acceptable to Jehovah's Witnesses have proved to be very effective and do not expose one to the hazards of blood transfusions. Christians know that only Jesus' shed blood is truly lifesaving. Faith in it brings forgiveness and the prospect of eternal life. – Ephesians 1:7."

[330] Organized to Accomplish Our Ministry, *supra* note 326, 171-3. Before baptism, congregation elders review with the prospective candidate basic Bible doctrine with the help of a series of questions and scriptures. If the candidate does not 'conform his life to Scriptural teachings', he will not be recommended for baptism (174). On the matter of blood, the following question and scriptures are discussed (191):

How do the following scriptures show that Jehovah considers blood as something sacred?

- Only flesh with its soul – its blood-you must not eat. – Genesis 9:4.
- Whenever your soul craves it you may slaughter, and you must eat meat according to the blessing of Jehovah your God....Only the blood you must not eat. On the earth you should pour it out as water. – Deuteronomy 12:15, 16.

It is noteworthy that Jehovah's Witnesses do not practice infant baptism.[331] Consequently, as in the process of conversion of new members, even children of Witness parents must be able to demonstrate that they understand Church doctrine and are decided to live in harmony with these principles before being baptized and formally accepted into the Witness faith.

The above may dispel the fears of the physician who perceives the Witness patient's refusal of blood therapy as an unreasoned allegiance to creed. That Church members consistently take the same firm position regarding the refusal of blood, even in life-threatening situations, argues that theirs is a premeditated and personal decision.

Their position on blood and blood fractions

The official position of Jehovah's Witnesses, as stated in their literature, is that "blood transfusions, whole blood, red cells, white cells, platelets, or blood plasma" are strictly forbidden by God's law. However, on the particular issue of "serum injections containing a tiny amount of a blood protein" such as "globulins,

---

- Any soul who eats any blood, that soul must be cut off from his people. – Leviticus 7:27.
- Keep abstaining from things sacrificed to idols, from blood and from things strangled. – Acts 15:29.
- Additional references: Leviticus 17:11; 1 Chronicles 11:18, 19; 1 Samuel 14:31-34; Romans 5:9.

Option questions for discussion:

a. How has the Scriptural view of blood affected your thinking on this matter?

b. As a Christian, what local foods or medical practices will you henceforth avoid?

c. How does the Bible teaching concerning the sanctity of life affect your view of certain dangerous sports or types of recreation?

d. Does God's view of life and blood seem reasonable to you?

e. What stand should a Christian take if he is told that in order to save his own life or the life of a loved one a blood transfusion would be needed?

See also Ridley, "Honoring Jehovah's Witnesses' Advance Directives in Emergencies: A Response to Drs Migden and Braen," 825.

[331] See "Should Babies Be Baptized?" The Watchtower, 7.

albumin, and fibrinogen" the acceptance of such treatment is left to the conscience of individual Witnesses. Consequently, while some members refuse blood fractions, others have conscientiously decided to accept such treatment, reasoning that "a tiny fraction of a donor's blood plasma ... used to bolster their defense against disease, is not the same as a life-sustaining blood transfusion," They also find some justification, amongst other things, in that during pregnancy "some protein fractions from the plasma do move naturally into the blood system" of the fetus.[332]

While transfusion of pre-stored autologous blood is ruled out, members decide personally whether or not to accept the use of hemodialysis devices (artificial kidney or heart-lung pump), induced hemodilution and blood salvage methods.[333] As evidenced in their openness to considering these types of devices and treatments, other than their conscientious objection to the use of blood, Jehovah's Witnesses "seek and accept standard medical treatment."[334]

---

332 "Questions from Readers," The Watchtower (1 June 1990), 31; "Questions from Readers," The Watchtower (15 June 2000), 30. The same article also states, "Should Christians accept these fractions in medical treatment? We cannot say. The Bible does not give details, so a Christian must make his own conscientious decision before God,." see also "Questions from Readers," The Watchtower (1 October 1994), 31; "Questions from Readers," The Watchtower (1 November 1961), 669; "Questions from Readers," The Watchtower (15 September 1958), 575. (This has been the position of *The Watchtower* for the last 40 years. On the matter of serums and vaccines containing blood fractions, it stated in 1958: "It would therefore be a matter of individual judgment whether one accepted such types of medication or not.")

333 "Questions from Readers," The Watchtower (15 October 2000), 30. Regarding the practice of preoperative autologous blood donation (PDA), the article stated, "However, such collecting, storing, and transfusion of blood directly contradicts what is said in Leviticus and Deuteronomy."; "Questions from Readers," The Watchtower (1 March 1959), 30. In deciding whether to permit the use of these methods, the Witness patient will want to know if their blood has been "poured out." For example, with the use of a hemodialysis device, patients may "view the external tubing as elongating their circulatory system so that blood might pass through an artificial organ. ... that the blood in this closed circuit was still part of them and did not need to be 'poured out'." The same reasoning may could apply to blood salvage methods which involve "circuit with recovery from a surgical site and ongoing reinfusion." These methods are also discussed in Spence, "Blood Management Policies for Jehovah's Witnesses," 148 & Joseph, Blood Conservation in the Surgical Patient, *supra* note 314 of chapter 3, 290-1; For early comments on the acceptability for Witnesses to accept blood salvage methods see "Questions from Readers," The Watchtower (15 October 1959), 640.

334 Spence, Clinical Practice of Transfusion Medicine, *supra* note 372, 602; Kitchens, "Are Transfusions Overrated? Surgical Outcome of Jehovah's Witnesses," 118.

The depth of their commitment

Jehovah's Witnesses are known to take their religion seriously. Health-care professionals have observed that with regards to the blood issue in particular, Jehovah's Witnesses "think deeply and pray earnestly about decisions regarding blood transfusion".[335] For them it is a religious decision for "(e)ven if doctors could give assurance that a transfusion would be totally safe, God's Word commands us to 'keep ourselves from blood.'"[336] Thus, to willfully accept a blood transfusion, whether directly or indirectly, means bearing personally "the responsibility for the violation of God's Law."[337] This is why, as stated by the Royal College of Surgeons of England, "Jehovah's Witnesses have absolutely refused the transfusion of blood and primary blood components ever since these techniques became universally available."[338]

The depth of commitment to their religious belief is seen from a resolution presented at their 1998 Annual District Assemblies held in major cities around the world and adopted by the thousands in attendance.[339] The resolution stated, among other things:

- We, as Jehovah's Witnesses assembled at the 'God's Way of Life' Convention, whole-heartedly agreed that God's way is the best way of life.

---

[335] Adams, "Respecting the Right to Be Wrong," *supra* note 267 of chapter 2, 753.

[336] "Be Faithful to God "Who Looks On in Secret", The Watchtower, 12.

[337] Rosam, "Patients' Rights and the Role of the Emergency Physician in the Management of Jehovah's Witnesses," 1151. Mr Rosam is writing as Director of Hospital Information Services at Jehovah's Witnesses international headquarters in Brooklyn, New York.

[338] The Royal College of Surgeons of England, Code of Practice for the Surgical Management of Jehovah's Witnesses, 1.

[339] For a partial report of these conventions see 1999 *Yearbook of Jehovah's Witnesses*, *supra* note 1, 7-16.

- We view ourselves as belonging to Jehovah God, having individually dedicated ourselves to him unconditionally, and we shall maintain unshakable faith in Jehovah's provision of the ransom through his Son, Jesus Christ.
- As individuals and as a religious organization, we will continue to put God's will first in our lives. Using his Word, the Bible, as our guide, we will not deviate to the right or to the left, thus confirming that God's way is far superior to the ways of the world.[340]

To impose a transfusion is a form of 'moral rape'

The Witness patient views an imposed or forced blood transfusion as "a gross physical violation"[341] equivalent to sexual assault.[342] One patient who learned that her objection to blood therapy had been ignored and a blood transfusion administered, described feeling "very, very dirty", as "if her privacy has been invaded and her body violated akin to sexual assault." Decrying the "severe emotional and mental upset" which had lasted for years, she agonized: "some days I don't feel like living."[343] Another young patient who went through the same experience expressed having felt "like a dog being used for an experiment."[344]

The physician who seeks to impose a blood transfusion can expect strong resistance from a conscious Witness patient. Even in the face of a court order, the patient will still consider a transfusion a "violation of God's law." If capable, the patient may attempt "to avoid being accessible" for the transfusion, even if this

---

340 "Keep on Walking in Jehovah's Way," The Watchtower, 19.

341 The Royal College of Surgeons of England, Code of Practice for the Surgical Management of Jehovah's Witnesses, *supra* note 338, 1.

342 "Questions from Readers," The Watchtower (15 June 1991), 31.

343 *Malette v. Shulmann & al., supra* note 269 of chapter 2, 274.

344 *Re L.D.K.; C.A.S. v. K.* (1985) 48 R.F.L. (2d) 164 (Ont. Prov. Ct.) Transcript of hearing at p. 28.

could lead to prosecution.[345] Physical resistance to a transfusion may include "screaming," "struggling," attempts to pull out "the injection device," even an effort "to destroy the blood bag."[346] This strong resistance is no doubt because their refusal "to consume blood is neither a mere ritual observance nor a minor dietary regulation; rather, it is a central expression of their relationship with God."[347]

Consequences of accepting or being forced to accept a transfusion

While Witnesses have long considered that "God's law requires that Christians abstain from blood, just as they are commanded to avoid fornication (sexual immorality),"[348] originally, congregations were not instructed to disfellowship or expel from their ranks those who voluntarily accepted blood transfusions. As it later developed however, members could face excommunication if found advocating an opposite view and to be unrepentant.[349] This measure was not however automatic.[350] To decide, congregation elders meet

---

345 "Questions from Readers," The Watchtower, *supra* note 342, 31. See also Rosam, "Patients' Rights and the Role of the Emergency Physician in the Management of Jehovah's Witnesses," *supra* note 337, 1151: "Whether an individual agrees to accept a blood transfusion or allows another authority to make this decision is immaterial. The individual still incurs the responsibility for the violation of God's law."

346 "Walk as Instructed by Jehovah," The Watchtower, 17.

347 Devine, "Save the Body, Lose the Soul," 68; Spence, "Management of Surgical Patients with Special Problems," *supra* note 372, 600. The author, who has treated many Jehovah's Witness patients describes his understanding of what would be the effect for one of these to accept a blood transfusion: "The consequences of transfusion for the Jehovah's Witness include excommunication from the church, forfeiture of a chance for eternal life, and severance of the individual's relationship with God."

348 "Questions from Readers," The Watchtower, *supra* note 342, 31.

349 "Questions from Readers," The Watchtower (15 January 1961), 63. "If, however, he refuses to acknowledge his nonconformity to the required Christian standard and makes the matter an issue in the Christian congregation and endeavors to influence others therein to his support; or, if in the future he persists in accepting blood transfusions or in donating blood toward the carrying out of this medical practice upon others, he shows that he has really not repented, but is deliberately opposed to God's requirements. As a rebellious opposer and unfaithful example to fellow members of the Christian congregation he must be cut off therefrom by disfellowshiping."

350 Malyon, "Transfusion-Free Treatment of Jehovah's Witnesses: Respecting the Autonomous Patient's Motives," *supra* note 281, 381.

as a 'judicial committee' with the individual with a view to 'recovery', to help 'the sinner readjust.' Only if it was determined that the person was guilty of 'remorseless apostasy, willful rebellion, or sheer wickedness' would 'disfellowshipping' occur.[351] However, since April 2000, members who voluntarily accept blood transfusions and openly advocate that position are simply deemed to have decided to cease being Jehovah's Witnesses.

Some writers have stated that "(a)mbivalent patients under stress may, in extremis, decide to accept transfusion or even indicate their wish to be coerced."[352] If and when this does happen, it seems to involve "newly acquainted" individuals.[353] Health-care professionals have observed, that, for the most part, "Jehovah's Witnesses have maintained a 'firm position' to 'absolutely refuse blood transfusion.'"[354] A survey in one of their congregations indicated that 58 out of 59 respondents would not consent to blood even if faced with death. One respondent answered '*probably* no.' In fact, the majority indicated that they would probably sue if administered a transfusion against their will. Interestingly, 46% had had bloodless surgery for themselves or a member of their family.[355]

---

[351] "Elders, Judge With Righteousness," The Watchtower, 19. The definition for disfellowshipping is: "dissociation or breaking off of spiritual fellowship and social intimacy." See "The Christian Congregation and Its Operation," The Watchtower, 600. Initially, congregations of Jehovah's Witnesses were not instructed to "disfellowship those who voluntarily take blood transfusions or approve them." See "Baptism," The Watchtower, 478.

[352] Macklin, "The Inner Workings of an Ethics Committee: Latest Battle over Jehovah's Witnesses," 16; Lang, Blood Conservation in the Surgical Patient, 328.

[353] "Be Faithful to God "Who Looks On in Secret," The Watchtower, 14 states: "Doctors and judges may try to persuade you to accept blood because they have seen people of other religions object to some medical step but then accept it 'behind close doors'. Some officials have even claimed to know of a Witness who agreed to a secret transfusion. *If* that did occur, it might have involved someone who was just acquainted with Jehovah's Witnesses."

[354] Andrews, "Legal, Ethical, and Medical Guidelines for Jehovah's Witnesses in Surgery," 1; The Royal College of Surgeons of England, Code of Practice for the Surgical Management of Jehovah's Witnesses, *supra* note 338, 1.

[355] Findley, "Blood Transfusion in Adult Jehovah's Witnesses, A Case Study of One Congregation," 606. See also Viele, "What Can We Learn About the Need For Transfusion From Patients Who Refuse Blood?," 396. From 1970 through to early 1993, Medline search reveals 4,722 cases of Jehovah's Witnesses who had refused blood transfusion therapy and were managed with alternatives. These do not include the statistical review by D. Cooley on 1,026 operations referred to in Dixon, "Blood: Whose Choice And Whose Conscience," 463.

There has been some question as to whether Witness patients administered a blood transfusion in spite their refusal are guilty of sin and would be ostracized by other members.[356] According to the Canadian director of HIS, in circumstances where an unauthorized transfusion is administered: "The person is offered psychological and emotional support, spiritual help and counseling. They are treated like a person who has been sexually assaulted, so they are offered assistance to cope. They are never ostracized, but are offered what they need most: support and encouragement."[357]

Jehovah's Witnesses believe that if they obey God's laws and exercise faith in Jesus Christ they will be rewarded with everlasting life on Earth transformed into a paradise under the rule of God's Kingdom.[358] As one author remarked, "understanding that the potential for everlasting life is an enormous incentive" with Jehovah's Witness patients will help the treating physician to understand his patient's adamant position against blood therapy.[359] Indeed to violate "such patients' deep and long-held religious convictions, the result could be tragic."[360] As observed by Pope John Paul II, forcing someone to violate his conscience "is the most painful blow inflicted to human dignity. In a certain sense, it is worse than inflicting physical death, or killing."[361]

---

[356] Macklin, "The Inner Workings of an Ethics Committee: Latest Battle over Jehovah's Witnesses," *supra* note 352, 16.

[357] Interview on 23 July 1999 with Mr Zenon Bodnaruk, Director of Hospital Information Services, Watch Tower Society, Canada Branch.

[358] Jehovah's Witnesses in the Twentieth Century, 13 for a detailed list of their beliefs.

[359] Spence, "Transfusion and Surgery," *supra* note 74, 1167.

[360] Dixon, "Blood: Whose Choice and Whose Conscience," *supra* note 354, 464.

[361] Quoted in Dixon, "Blood: Whose Choice and Whose Conscience," *supra* note 354, 464.

Section 2

ETHICAL AND LEGAL ISSUES RAISED BY THE OBJECTION

5. New Principles and Rules

There was a time when the doctor was "as it were, alone with his patient and God." [362] The end of the post Second World War period brought about important changes in health-care that would revolutionize this doctor-patient relationship. Technology and specialization moved in. The individual physician, alone at the bedside of his patient, gave way to teams of highly specialized doctors working with sophisticated technical equipment in modern hospitals. This led to "the altered social position of medicine … with the fact that the doctor became a stranger and the hospital a strange place."[363] New rules were needed as patient and doctor became 'strangers at the bedside' and did not always share the same values. One author states: "When one could no longer assume that the physician shared the same set of values as the patient, it seemed vital to devise and implement new mechanisms, preferably formal or even rigid, to further patients' particular wishes. It became appropriate to post on hospital walls a copy of the Patient Bill of Rights."[364]

In light of these changes, it became necessary to reassess the 'Hippocratic ethic.'[365] As a result 'medical ethics' or 'bioethics' emerged as a guiding light to

---

362 Jonas, "Philosophical Reflections on Experimenting with Human Subjects," 238.

363 Rothman, Strangers at the Bedside, 11.

364 Rothman, Strangers at the Bedside, *supra* note 363, 11.

365 Pellegrino, Hippocrates Revisited A Search for Meaning, 134. The Hippocratic ethic refers to 'admonitions found scattered throughout the Hippocratic corpus' which form 'a mixture of high ideals, common sense, and practical wisdom.'

help doctors and patients reestablish a meaningful relationship of mutual trust and respect. "Ethics is the enterprise of disciplined reflection on the moral intuitions and moral choices that people make. Medical ethics is the analysis of choices made in the medical sphere. Medical ethics covers choices made not only by physicians, but also by other health professionals – nurses, pharmacists, hospital chaplains, and so forth. More important, it covers choices made by medical lay people – patients, parents, legislators, public officials, and judges."[366]

Bioethics, or *medical ethics* as used in the context of problem-solving in clinical practice, is a process of logical enquiry into what actions are right or wrong. This process will usually lead to a consideration of principles and values relevant to the treatment of a patient that affect the doctor-patient relationship. Such principles and values may include the 'life is sacred' principle, autonomy, paternalism and informed consent. While the process will rarely produce a sole comprehensive answer to a given problem, it may help guide the physician treating a patient.[367]

Also, with an educated public, "the notion of the physician as a benevolent and paternalistic who decides all for the patient" became outmoded.[368] The physician now encountered knowledgeable patients who expected the doctor to be "alert to (his) responsibility in the relationship, just as you would in any other

---

[366] For a definition of ethics in the medical context see: Veatch, Medical Ethics, 1. Regarding the term bioethics, Veatch writes at p. 6: "Sometimes the term *bioethics* is used instead of medical ethics. The terms are now used almost interchangeable. Sometimes bioethics has a slightly broader meaning, including ethical problems of the biological sciences outside of medicine – research on animals, efforts to manipulate the genetic makeup of nonhuman species, and so forth."

[367] Health Sciences Ethics Education Committee, Introduction to Ethical Decision-Making in Health Care, 1: "Ethics as a theoretical discipline is a formal, scholarly, logical enquiry into what actions are good or right (that is, moral) and why certain actions are good or right. Applied to clinical practice it leads to action based on rules, principles, and values, and seeks to resolve conflicts of value that arise in the course of treating patients. While ethics may not always come up with a single or simple solution to problems arising in clinical practice, it serves to clarify the practitioner's thinking and to facilitate making ethical decisions in an orderly way rather than on an ad hoc basis."

[368] Pellegrino, Hippocrates Revisited A Search for Meaning, *supra* note 365, 135.

adult relationship where you are purchasing services."[369] When exercising their right to medical decision-making, formerly 'powerless patients' now found support in the movement toward a commitment to bioethics.[370] According to D. Rothman: "In the end, the initial commitment of bioethics to patients' rights helps account for its extraordinary accomplishments in the decade from 1966 to 1976. The fit between the movement and the times was perfect. Just when courts were defining an expanded right to privacy, the bioethicists were emphasizing the principle of autonomy, and the two meshed neatly; judges supplied a legal basis and bioethicists a philosophical basis for empowering the patient. Indeed, just when movements on behalf of a variety of minorities were advancing their claims, the bioethicists were defending another group that appeared powerless – patients."

As a result of this transition, "informed and empowered patients" began to "serve as active and skilled partners in managing their own health."[371]

These were major changes in health-care that attempted to level the playing field in the doctor-patient relationship. New principles and rules emerged and these had a direct impact on patients who disagree with recommended treatment by physicians.

Notwithstanding these changes, Jehovah's Witness patients who refuse to consent to the use of blood products in their treatment have continued to prove to be a real challenge to the medical community. Since, as observed by one physician, "the true Jehovah's Witness cannot be dissuaded" from this position, it has been difficult at times for some physicians to deal with the Witness' objection

---

369 Haug, "Practitioner or Patient – Who's in Charge?" 215

370 Rothman, Strangers at the Bedside, *supra* note 363, 245.

371 These comments were published by the National Health Council, a nonprofit American association of 118 national health organizations dedicated to accessible health care for patients. Information about them as well as their official booklet is posted on the web at: http://www.healthanswers.com/Sources/nhc/ppf.html; See also Carlson, "Patient Representatives Aid Physicians, Too," 34. This article shows the expanding role of patient representatives or advocates aiding patients to "become successful partners in their own care."

to blood transfusion.[372] This has sometimes resulted in "confusion" on the part of health-care professionals and "emotional bias" against the Witness patient.[373] A contributing factor may be that from medical school on the physician is taught that blood transfusion saves lives; thus a refusal will often be deemed unreasonable and tantamount to suicide. Many doctors sincerely feel they are prevented from respecting the maxim *primum non nocere*, if they are not given the opportunity to administer blood.

However, such 'confusion' and conflict can and should be avoided. Principles and rules which at first sight may seem to some conflicting can in effect work together to protect the patient's autonomy while respecting the physician's obligation 'to do no harm.'

---

[372] Spence, Clinical Practice of Transfusion Medicine, 600.

[373] Minuck & Lambie, "Anesthesia and Surgery for Jehovah's Witnesses," 1187.

6. 'Life is Sacred' Principle

Life-saving or not?

Our brief historical review of the use of blood in medicine revealed that the practice has often been enshrouded with mysticism and ignorance. Convinced of its' life giving 'magical' properties, some bathed in blood while others drank it, hoping for a cure.[374] Bloodletting, or phlebotomy, became standard treatment for centuries, only to fall into disrepute and eventually give way to blood transfusion therapy. Through it all, blood was always the "queen of remedies" with near 'magical' properties. As blood transfusion became standard medical practice, little attention was given to the dangers surrounding it until the catastrophic events in the 1980s involving tainted blood. Since then, a more measured approach to the use of blood therapy has been encouraged and more and more patients are looking for alternatives.[375]

Nevertheless, blood transfusion remains a standard medical therapy and is probably one of the most readily prescribed procedures today. Physicians in general continue to regard it as 'life-saving' in many situations.[376] They argue that without it, surgery in many cases would be impossible, hemophiliacs would die and many trauma patients would not survive.[377] Blood collection agencies

---

[374] *Supra* note 92 and accompanying text.

[375] Thomas, "Nonblood Management in Obstetrics and Gynecology," *supra* note 310, 475.

[376] That blood continues to be considered the gift of life by many can be seen by the comments of author Andre Picard who, after recounting the horrors of the Canadian blood scandal and considering numerous infectious agents known to be blood-borne, went on to write: "None of this is intended to create a panic, or to scare people who really need transfusions away from accepting blood. Blood truly is the Gift of Life to accident and burn victims, and many major surgery patients; we can't lose sight of that." Picard, The Gift of Death, *supra* note 167 of chapter 2, 232.

[377] Spence, Blood and Blood Products: Safety and Risk, *supra* note 170, 87-91. "Thus transfusion is still a major part of coronary bypass surgery. ... (W)e still need allogeneic blood to make these kinds of procedures possible. ... Other areas of medicine that would not be possible today without transfusion include level I trauma centers. ... (P)atients with hemophilia and the inherent coagulopathies would all

counter the fallout from negative media coverage of the tainted blood disaster by stressing the continued need for blood to 'save lives,' often using children as spokespersons.[378] Most health-care professionals consider blood transfusion, "a simple form of treatment." Individuals, who on religious or moral grounds refuse blood recommended by the physician, will often be perceived as unreasonable and irrational by attending health-care personnel who believe that such refusal "may lead directly to their death."[379]

Yet, to consider blood as only a 'simple form of treatment', and its refusal as a decision often leading to death, is to ignore the intricacies of a complex human organism and the serious hazards associated with the practice of transfusing it.[380] Administering blood transfusion does not necessarily mean 'saving a life' and refusing one does not necessarily mean 'death.' As stated by one author: "Blood is usually administered by physicians with the nearly unchallenged view that failure to transfuse would have dire consequences. Evidence supporting that view is difficult to obtain."[381] In addition, the death of thousands of patients who accepted blood transfusions during the tainted blood crisis speaks against equating the refusal of blood transfusions to suicide.

A fact unknown to many is that there exists little or no scientific data by which to evaluate the overall appropriate use of blood products.[382] Some health-care professionals have pointed to the "surprising, even appalling, lack of

---

die at young ages."

378 During the summer months of 1999, *HEMA Québec,* blood agency for the province, carried on an extensive media campaign using mainly young children in a drive to obtain blood donations.

379 Gilmartin, Ethical Issues in Anaesthesia, 103. Here the author is oversimplifying: "The particular problem posed by Jehovah's Witnesses is that their refusal of a relatively simple form of treatment may lead directly to their death."

380 See *supra* notes 241, 242 and 243.

381 Kitchens, "Are Transfusions Overrated? Surgical Outcome of Jehovah's Witnesses," *supra* note 334, 117.

382 US. Congress, Office of Technology Assessment Task Force, Blood Technologies, Services, and Issues, 121.

adequate studies on the value of and indications for blood products."[383] *The Lancet* reported: "Despite more than five decades of established practice, doctors still do not agree about precisely when and why they should transfuse red cells and how efficacy can be assessed. .... For most areas of surgical practice the lack of incontrovertible proof of benefit from red-cell transfusion, despite subjective impressions, might seem disquieting. After all, what widely available drug could be used under such imprecise circumstances?"[384]

Reports and surveys indicate that in many cases physicians have little or no scientific knowledge to rely on when ordering transfusions, yet they do so with the "greatest confidence."[385] Thus, according to the U.S. Congress Office of Technology Assessment Task Force "the practice at the bedside relies on anecdotal reports and evidence from inadequate trials."[386]

While it is important to take into account these more questionable aspects of blood therapy, the case being considered is that of the patient whose objection to the use of blood is based on religious or moral grounds. Whether or not it 'saves lives' is of secondary importance to the individual who believes that accepting a blood transfusion is a grave violation of God's law.

Sanctity of life principle

The issue of 'life saving' treatment evokes the 'sanctity of life' principle. While this principal permeates the medical ethics debate, its' meaning remains

---

383 Ellison & Silberstein, A Commentary on Three Consensus Development Conferences on Transfusion Medicine, 609, 624.

384 Napier, Towards More Rational Use of Red Cells, The Lancet, 1280.

385 Salem-Schatz, Influence of Clinical Knowledge, Organizational Context, and Practice Style on Transfusion Decision Making, 479, 482; Stehling, A Survey of Transfusion Practices Among Anesthesiologists, 60-2; US. Congress, Office of Technology Assessment Task Force, Blood Technologies, Services, and Issues, *supra* note 382, 128.

386 US. Congress, Office of Technology Assessment Task Force, Blood Technologies, Services, and Issues, *supra* note 382, 127.

"open to innumerable differences in interpretation."[387] As an example, in the conflict that can often oppose patient and physician on the issue of refusing a blood transfusion, both sides, paradoxically, substantiate their position by referring to the 'sanctity of life' principle. On the one hand, the Jehovah's Witness patient argues that in the Bible God forbids humans to consume the "lifeblood" (Genesis 9:3-6). "Blood had a special meaning. It stood for life provided by the Creator." Both life and blood are considered 'holy' or sacred. Taking the position that "those who respect life as a gift from the Creator do not try to sustain it by taking in blood" for to do so would be "unholy," the Witness disavows accepting blood as a violation of the 'sanctity of life' principle.[388] On the other hand, the physician opposes such a refusal on the premise that blood 'saves lives', it is the very 'gift of life', and "because human life is at stake, every reasonable attempt ought to be made to save that life."[389] For the physician, being denied the opportunity to administer blood to 'save a life' is a violation of the 'sanctity of life' principle. Which argument is correct, and who decides?

Religious and secular viewpoints

While the 'life is sacred' principle is implicitly present in Eastern religions and in Judeo-Christian and Hippocratic traditions, an extensive literature review failed to identify explicit pre-twentieth-century references to this principle.[390] One of the earlier references applying the principle outside religious discourse is less than half a century old and is found in Glanville Williams' work entitled *The*

---

[387] Callahan, The Sanctity of Life, 185.

[388] How Can Blood Save Your Life?, *supra* note 5 of chapter 1, 4, 6 and 25. See also *supra* note 19 of chapter 1 and accompanying text.

[389] Green, "Biblical Laws Relating to Blood Transfusion: The Judaic Laws and Principles," *supra* note 281 of chapter 3, 247.

[390] Khushf, Sanctity of Life and Human Dignity, 294.

Sanctity of Life and the Criminal Law.[391]

From a *religious* viewpoint, the life is sacred principle generally "bespeaks life to be God's creation, over which we have no authority; life is a gift-in-trust from God, and we are pledged to practice good stewardship of it; it is for our use, but it is only on loan."[392] Expressed differently: "Every human being is a unique, unrepeatable opportunity to praise God. His life is entirely an ordination, a loan, and a stewardship."[393] From this same religious standpoint, each of "us is created in the image or likeness of God" and our behavior must "mirror in some way the divine glory."[394] For those who adopt this approach, humans received their worth and dignity entirely from God and, as a result, their life is sacred.[395]

However, not all proponents of the 'sanctity of life' principle are believers in God. Some approach the issue from a different angle, from a *secular* point of view, hoping to reach a larger audience.[396] They point "to the nature of things, to the way things are, a protoreligious, natural metaphysic."[397] Sacredness is

---

[391] Williams, The Sanctity of Life and Criminal Law.

[392] Clouser, "The Sanctity of Life: An Analysis of a Concept," 119.

[393] Ramsey, Moral Problems: A Collection of Philosophical Essays, 11.

[394] Sevensky, "The Religious Foundations of Health Care: A Conceptual Approach," 165. Those who adopt this viewpoint also believe that human life begins at the moment of conception. See Koop, "The Sanctity of Life," 62.

[395] In Keyserlingk, Sanctity of Life or Quality of Life, 13, after a thorough discussion, the following conclusions are drawn from the religious viewpoint of the 'Quality of life' principle:

(i) The sanctity of human life is not the result of the "worth" a human being may attribute to it – either to one's own life or that of others. Considerations such as "degrees of relative worth," "functional proficiency," or "pragmatic utility" which humans may acquire or have are in no sense appropriate yardsticks for determining or measuring sanctity of life.

(ii) Human life may not be taken without adequate justification, nor may human nature be radically changed.

(iii) The sanctity of life principle is basic to our society, and its rejection would endanger all human life.

[396] Since the study of ethics is to "seek that to which all rational men could agree," the religious viewpoint is considered by many to be too limited in our modern pluralistic society. "Generally, religious requirements are more stringent than what could be expected of all rational men. They go beyond the reasonable obligation, beyond the call of duty; they require you to go the second mile." See Clouser, "The Sanctity of Life: An Analysis of a Concept," *supra* note 392, 119.

[397] Keyserlingk, Sanctity of Life or Quality of Life, *supra* note 395, 14.

inherent to humans because they are alive and conscious. "The idea of sacredness is generated by the primordial experience of being alive, of experiencing the elemental sensation of vitality and the elemental fear of its extinction."[398] Of course, such an explanation begs a definition for 'sacredness' used in the non-religious context: is it a property, a feeling, a value, a right or simply an overall life orientation? One writer concludes from such an analysis that "the sanctity of life concept as it is generally used – not in its original religious sense – is only a slogan."[399]

For some, this secular viewpoint is more accurately described as a *qualified* 'sanctity of life' principle.[400] While conceding that it is "elusive and indeterminate," some authors have portrayed it in the following way: "It *does* point to an objective, absolute value of human life and worth, it insists that human life is always worthy of respect and protection, and that it should always be supported without adequate justification to the contrary."[401]

The application of the 'sanctity of life' principle, whether religious or secular, has sometimes promoted 'vitalism', that is the concept that advocates "preservation of human life, even mere metabolism and vital processes, no matter what the patient's condition."[402] This view of the 'sanctity of life' principle held by some health-care professionals and judges kept patients such as Karen Quinlan and Nancy Cruzan in a 'persistent vegetative state' for years.

In 1975, Karen Ann Quinlan, a 21-year-old, suffered brain damage after swallowing alcohol and tranquilizers at a party. After hospitalization, it was determined that the damage was irreversible and that she was in a persistent

---

[398] Shils, Life or Death: Ethics and Options, 12-13.

[399] Sevensky, "The Religious Foundations of Health Care: A Conceptual Approach," *supra* note 394, 124.

[400] Kuhse, The Sanctity-of-Life Doctrine in Medicine, 23.

[401] Keyserlingk, Sanctity of Life or Quality of Life, *supra* note 395, 49.

[402] *Ibid.*, 19.

vegetative state. The family requested the removal of the life-support system (respirator) which they deemed to be 'extraordinary means,' but the primary-care physician refused. It became necessary for the family to petition the courts. They lost at trial, but won in the New Jersey Supreme Court.[403] However, by that time, Karen had been weaned off the respirator and although breathing on her own, was still being kept alive with artificially provided nutrition and hydration. Evidently, the family did not consider these artificial measures to be 'extraordinary means' since they did not request that this form of life support be terminated. Karen remained in her 'persistent vegetative state' until her death eight years later.

A few years later, in 1983, following a car accident, Nancy Beth Cruzan was kept in a "persistent vegetative state" for seven years while her family fought through the courts for permission to let her die.[404] Judging artificial hydration and nutrition to be extraordinary means, they petitioned the court to have them withdrawn. While the trial court agreed with the family's petition, the attorney general of the State of Missouri argued successfully in the Missouri Supreme Court that the state's interest in preserving Nancy's life, regardless of the quality of her life, outweighed her right to refuse treatment. The Supreme Court of United States, for its part, required from the family clear and convincing evidence that it was the patient's desire to have hydration and nutrition withdrawn. Following the Supreme Court's decision, the family presented such evidence to the courts and obtained permission to stop feeding her; Nancy died 12 days later.

Through long and difficult legal battles such as these, and following numerous confrontations between doctors and members of patients' families, it became evident that vitalism, or the preservation of 'life' regardless of the patient's condition was not morally defendable. Today, vitalism in medical

---

[403] *Matter of Quinlan*, 70 N.J. 10 (1976) Supreme Court of New Jersey.

[404] *Cruzan, by her parents and co-Guardians v. Director, Missouri Department of Health, Supreme Court of the United States*, 497 U.S. 261, June 25, 1990, decided.

decision-making has few supporters.[405]

A more temperate view suggests that the *qualified* (or *secular*) 'sanctity of life' principle be used to test particular moral rules; an "indeterminate ethical principle to judge and test determinate rules of conduct."[406] This may be a useful approach since "principles and rules appear to remain central in biomedical ethics."[407] Viewed this way the 'sanctity of life' principle implies a spectrum of values ranging from the preservation of the species to the inviolability of human bodies, from man in the aggregate (present and future) to man as an individual (present and future).[408] The *qualified* 'sanctity of life' principle, with the corollary 'principles and rules' applicable to the situation of the conscientious objector to medical treatment, is the approach that will be adopted in the present analysis.[409]

Furthermore, this analysis must take into account the specific viewpoint on the 'sanctity of life' principle held by the particular group or individual objecting, on moral or religious grounds, to a recommended medical treatment. Views may vary according to the individual or group. Citing religious principles, a Catholic may refuse to proceed with a recommended abortion, while someone of the Jewish or Muslim faith may invoke religious belief in refusing a recommended surgery or treatment involving porcine products. A careful analysis of those varying viewpoints will be essential if the doctor is to proceed in a manner that does not violate the deeply held beliefs of the patient. In the case under study, this will involve analyzing the *religious* viewpoint of Jehovah's Witnesses.

---

405 Kuhse, The Sanctity-of-Life Doctrine in Medicine, *supra* note 400, 199.

406 Keyserlingk, Sanctity of Life or Quality of Life, *supra* note 395, 42.

407 Childress, Medical Ethics, 52.

408 Callahan, The Sanctity of Life, *supra* note 387, 208.

409 It has been said though, that the debate over the 'sanctity of life' issue is "the most controversial and complex medical and ethical issue" facing both the health profession and society in general. There are no 'simple and elegant solutions to the problem.' See Gilmore, "Sanctity of Life Versus Quality of Life – The Continuing Debate," 181.

Sanctity of life – Jehovah's Witnesses' viewpoint

Jehovah's Witnesses consider human life as sacred, a gift from their Creator. To support this, they point to the Bible statement: "For with you (God) is the fountain of life."[410] For them, (r)espect for life is a sacred obligation to the "Giver of life, Jehovah God."[411] They believe that their life does not belong to them, "but is only entrusted to us by God."[412] For this reason, they encourage their members to "cultivate appreciation for life as a gift from God" by maintaining a lifestyle that is conducive to good health.[413] This would include leading a healthy lifestyle and avoiding excesses that "can be instrumental in shortening the life-span. In this classification would fall alcoholism, drug addiction and over nutrition."[414]

Considering life as sacred, they prohibit the use of tobacco.[415] Reckless driving, extreme sports and any form of negligence that puts lives in danger are strongly discouraged.[416] They are not in favor of having abortions[417] and suicide is not an option.[418] Even in the case of great suffering and terminal illness, they

---

410 Psalm 36:9.

411 True Peace and Security – How Can You Find It?, 152-3.

412 "Treasure the Real Life," The Watchtower, 6.

413 True Peace and Security – How Can You Find It?, *supra* note 411, 152. This would include avoiding a "promiscuous course that often leads to death." See "How Precious Is Life to You?" The Watchtower, 3.

414 "Doing What We Can to Maintain a Better Life," Awake!, 6.

415 "Keeping God's Congregation Clean in the Time of His Judgment," The Watchtower, 339: "Tobacco's damaging effect on the body is well known and its befouling effect is just as evident. Surely it does not show respect for the Creator having given us life if we misuse and befoul our bodies through tobacco addiction."

416 "How Precious is Life to You?" The Watchtower, 3; "Thrill Sports – Should I Take a Chance?" Awake!, 9 (extreme sports); "Motorcycles – How Dangerous Are They?" Awake!, 10 (dangers of high speed motorcycles); "Bullfighting – Art or Outrage?" Awake!, 19 (bullfighting); "Water Safety Is No Accident," Awake!, 15 (negligence in water sports).

417 "Questions from Readers," The Watchtower (15 March 1975), 191.

418 "Why the Rise in Suicide?" Awake!, 25. With regards to God's judgment of those who do commit suicide, they make the following comment: "But the living may be absolutely confident that He is also merciful and understanding. He alone knows all the complex personal and social factors that can torment an otherwise healthy person into believing he must kill himself. The Bible shows that 'the

do not advocate active euthanasia.

All this, however, does not mean that where a person is suffering greatly from a disease and death is only a matter of time that a physician must continue to take extraordinary, complicated, distressing and costly measures to keep the patient alive. There is a great difference between extending the life of a patient and stretching out the dying process. In such cases it would not be violating God's law regarding the sanctity of life to mercifully let the dying process take its due course. The medical profession generally acts in harmony with this principle.[419]

While Jehovah's Witnesses attach great importance to their temporal life, they believe that the 'true life' is the promised future – eternal life. They base this reasoning on the Bible text of 1 Timothy 6:17-19 which states in part: "(T)hey will lay up treasure for themselves as a firm foundation for the coming age, so that they may take hold of the life that is truly life." Verse 12 of the same chapter states: "Fight the good fight of the faith. Take hold of the eternal life to which you were called when you made your good confession in the presence of may witnesses." For Witnesses, 'eternal life' means that God-fearing humans can look forward to life everlasting on Earth transformed into a paradise under the heavenly reign of Jesus Christ as king of God's Kingdom.[420] They believe that to attain this they must exercise faith in the ransom sacrifice of Jesus Christ and be baptized.

Judge of all the earth is going to do what is right.' – Genesis 18:25"

[419] "Euthanasia and God's Law," The Watchtower, 118. This article points to the example of Job (Job 2: 4-10) who "suffered greatly from a very loathsome disease as well as from many misfortunes" yet he remained faithful to God during his suffering. Witnesses believe that suffering does not justify violating the sanctity of life principle through euthanasia. They state that "God's word plainly tells that human life is sacred and that he who takes a human life must forfeit his own." "Mercy Killing – What Do Lawyers Say?" Awake!, 7.

[420] They also believe a selected few, that is 144,000, will resurrect for 'eternal life' with Christ in his heavenly kingdom. See Knowledge That Leads to Everlasting Life, *supra* note 8, chapter 10, "God's Kingdom Rules," 90-7.

While they do not believe that baptism is a sacrament,[421] they hold the view that through baptism they dedicate their lives to God and undertake to do his will.[422] This includes adhering to various Bible principles. Two of these principles are: refusing to participate in wars and refusing to accept blood transfusions or blood products.[423] They adhere to these two positions because of what the 'life is sacred' principle means to them. Their Bible trained conscience, which has prompted them to take a firm stand on these issues, has at times put them at odds not only with medical personnel, but also with political authorities.

For example, during the Second World War, Hitler harshly punished German nationals who did not support his war effort. Rebuffing an enraged Hitler, Jehovah's Witnesses in Germany refused all participation in military service. As a result, during the war about 10,000 Jehovah's Witnesses were imprisoned and an estimated 2,500 to 5,000 died.[424] For them, obedience to God on the issue of 'sacredness of life' had a higher value than their temporal life. Their position was non-negotiable even though many were offered freedom in return for apposing a simple signature to a document stating they renounced their faith.[425] This was really a question of loyalties and principles. If they were loyal to Hitler, they would go to war and be ready to take the lives of others and

---

421 "Should You be Baptized?" The Watchtower, 4, 6: "The Scriptures do not support that widely held religious view that baptism is a sacrament, that is, a religious ceremony imparting merit – grace, holiness, or spiritual benefit – to the one baptized."

422 "Gaining Peace With God Through Dedication and Baptism," The Watchtower, 12.

423 By not participating in wars they believe they are upholding "the sanctity of blood, of human life and also the standard for God's people to 'beat their swords into plowshares and not learn war anymore.' See "Facing Up to Questions of Conscience," The Watchtower, 589. They also believe that "to go out on the battlefield and slaughter their fellow believers of another country" would be contrary to Jesus' words: "By this all men will know that you are my disciples, if you love one another." (John 13:35) See You Can Live Forever in Paradise on Earth, *supra* note 23, 189.

424 Information obtained at the United States Holocaust Memorial Museum in a pamphlet entitled *Jehovah's Witnesses*. See also Graffard, Les Bibelforscher et le nazisme (1933-1945) Ces oubliés de l'Histoire.

425 During the Second World War, Witnesses were also imprisoned in several countries for refusing military service including Canada, United States and Australia. However, in these latter countries they were neither tortured nor executed while in prison, contrary to Germany. See Kaplan, State and Salvation, 190-223.

possibly lose their own life on the battlefield. But, if they were loyal to their God Jehovah, they must then refuse military service, although for many of them it would mean torture and execution. In the latter case they would have prized their future 'eternal life' and the life of their fellowman more than their own present life. They would have lived according to the dictates of their conscience as to the sacredness of life. Jehovah's Witnesses continue to be conscientious objectors to military service in all countries down to this day.[426]

Their position regarding blood transfusions is similarly "non-negotiable".[427] They take the position that "(t)hose who respect life as a gift from the Creator do not try to sustain life by taking in blood" in contravention to his commandments.[428] Judging by the Witnesses' proven stalwart refusal to participate in war, physicians can expect an equally adamant rejection of blood transfusions.

Quality of life argument

Before broaching the aspect of 'principles and rules' which has a direct bearing on this discussion (autonomy and informed consent), it would be helpful to briefly address the 'quality of life' concept, since "the sanctity of life principle is not by itself concrete and determinate enough to answer all questions."[429] Some argue that the "marriage of these two concepts" may be possible if extreme views of each are abandoned.[430]

---

426 See for example the story of Fernando Marin who spent 10 years (1964-1973) in a Spanish jail for refusing military service in "My Ten Year s in Spain's Military Prisons," The Watchtower, 19.

427 How Can Blood Save Your Life?, *supra* note 5 of chapter 1, 6.

428 *Ibid.*

429 Keyserlingk, Sanctity of Life or Quality of Life, *supra* note 395, 50. According to D. Callahan, reference to the quality of life criteria poses certain problems. "The problem I think is that quality of life is a systematically ambiguous concept and thus I see it as a conceptual, unguided missile likely to be used in any and all ways by different people with no particular agreement on proper usage." See Gilmore, "Sanctity of Life Versus Quality of Life – The Continuing Debate," *supra* note 409, 180.

430 D. Callahan recommends a "move away from extreme views of the sanctity of life and quality of life.

The sanctity of life principle requires *justifiable* reasons for ceasing to preserve human life. As stated by Kuhse: "Despite this widespread theoretical commitment to the sanctity of all human life, there are, however, ultimately few people (if any) who will follow where their theory should logically lead them – namely, to the preservation of all human lives, irrespective of the quality of those lives."[431]

This means that there should be some consensus, at least, that other considerations be examined. Certainly in the health-care context, one of these considerations must be the quality of life criterion. In applying the quality of life criterion, it should be remembered that the sanctity of life principal considers *all* persons as having intrinsic worth and of equal value. To treat patients otherwise could render the practitioner guilty of narrowing he view only "to what science can reveal about them" and "objectifying and diminishing" them to simple "things to be managed."[432] In view of this, it would seem necessary to exclude considerations "such as social worth, social utility, social status or relative worth" and concentrate on the "objective improvement or reduction of discomfort or some other benefit" to the patient.[433] It would be very difficult, even "impossible

He suggest that the greatest obstacle to the marriage of these two concepts is the lack of agreement on the meaning of the notion of quality." See Gilmore, "Sanctity of Life Versus Quality of Life – The Continuing Debate," *supra* note 409, 180. In his final proposals to the Canadian Law Reform Commission, Keyserlingk blesses the marriages between these two principles as follows: "Public policy and law should (continue to) affirm and protect the absolute value, equality and "sanctity" of human life, (...). But at the same time, it should make explicit that what it is affirming and protecting is the absolute value of human *personal* life, of persons." (...) "Applied to both competent and incompetent patients the determinative criterion is the *patient's perspective*, the patient's benefit." See Keyserlingk, Sanctity of Life or Quality of Life, *supra* note 395, 187.

431 See Kuhse, "The Quality/Quantity-of-Life Distinction and its Moral Importance for Nurses," 205: "Amongst medical professionals the practice of allowing some hopelessly or incurably ill patients to die is near-universal (Singer & al., 1983) and a closer look at the writings of theologians and philosophers who regard themselves as champions of the sanctity-of-life view, reveals that they typically make implicit or covert quality-of-life judgments.

432 Gillett, "Learning to Do No Harm," 264.

433 Keyserlingk proposes this restricted or more qualified meaning of quality of life in response to proponents of the principal who would "welcome the replacement of the "traditional" ethics of the absolute value of human life by an ethic of its relative value and in response to opponents who fear that "any recognition of quality of life factors" is a danger to the "intrinsic worth and equal value of

to determine what will benefit a patient without presupposing some quality-of-life standard and some conception of the life the patient will live after a medical intervention."[434] In this sense, the quality of life criterion will focus on what is beneficial to the patient, what is in the 'best interests' of the patient. This will have particular application to incompetent patients on whose behalf others must decide. Of course, any advance directives by the patient will have an important bearing on the quality of life analysis. This will be discussed further on.

For the competent patient, the quality of life criterion will be subjective, determined by the patient, and only the patient, since the right to accept or refuse medical treatment in this case is well established both legally and morally. "That clearly and unequivocally establishes a "hands off" policy as regards to *anyone* interfering with that right and imposing treatment for any reason whatsoever."[435] This is reasonable as the competent patient has the best vantage point to decide what is in his or her best interest, whether others agree with the decision or not.

This brings the discussion to the principle of autonomy, a principle that recognizes the right of patients to self-determination. In cases where a competent patient refuses what is deemed to be life-saving medical treatment, does the exercise of self-determination violate the 'sanctity of life' principle? If, as discussed above, the quality of life criterion is applied when addressing the sanctity of life issue, then the logical conclusion should be that a patient's autonomy must be respected since only the patient can decide what treatment is morally acceptable to him.

---

every human." The ultimate aim of the quality of life criteria "is objective improvement and benefit, even if ... that will often be limited to reducing rather than eliminating the patient's discomfort and dignity." Keyserlingk, Sanctity of Life or Quality of Life, *supra* note 395, 51-3, 59.

[434] Beauchamp, Principles of Biomedical Ethics, 216.

[435] Keyserlingk, Sanctity of Life or Quality of Life, *supra* note 395, 112.

7. The Principle of Autonomy

No man is good enough to treat another without his consent.

P. Ramsey[436]

To recognize a person as autonomous is to respect him, to give him dignity. According to Immanuel Kant, a person's dignity, his sublimity, comes from being morally autonomous.[437] People possess an autonomous, self-legislating will that confers upon them intrinsic worth and dignity. Kant's theory focuses on the individual's unconditional worth and his capacity to determine his own destiny. For John Stewart Mill, a society cannot really be free if it does not recognize the right of an individual to "do as he likes," as long as he does not harm others. He argues that whether the individual's conduct is popular or not, whether it is foolish or not, is irrelevant and that person must be protected "against the tyranny of the prevailing opinion and feeling."[438]

The notion of autonomy is not limited to certain aspects of one's life. On the contrary, it encompasses the whole person as he lives out his life. As expressed by one writer: "The right to control one's body means not only the right to defend oneself against the outside world. It also involves and even primarily refers to a person's right to decide freely and sovereignly on the course of his own life. Freedom, which is essential and basic to human dignity, consists foremost in the freedom to act and live in accordance with one's social, philosophical and religious ideas."[439][translation]

---

436 Ramsey, The Patient as a Person, 137.

437 Kant, Immanuel Kant, Practical Philosophy, 85.

438 Mill, Essential Works of John Stuart Mill, 285.

439 Dierkens, Les droits sur le corps et le cadavre de l'homme, 42.

Respect for the individual's right to autonomy, in health-care as well as in other aspects of life, is an integral part of the very fabric of the modern democratic society. As stated recently by the Supreme Court of Canada: "All individuals have the right to make personal decisions, to control their bodily integrity, and to refuse unwanted medical treatment. These are not mere legal technicalities; they represent some of the *most deeply held values in society* and form the *basis* for fundamental and constitutional human rights."[440] [Emphasis added]

Respect for autonomy is thus not only a legal obligation but also a moral one "in so far as such respect is compatible with equal respect for the autonomy of all potentially affected."[441] Consequently, one cannot invoke autonomy to violate the autonomy of others. The classic example of a person mendaciously yelling "fire" in a crowded theater and needlessly putting people's lives in danger illustrates that there are situations where an individual's autonomy can rightly be restricted both morally and legally.

In health-care situations a person's right to self-determination could easily be violated. These circumstances necessitate the conscientious application of the principle of autonomy and its many implications such as the need for informed consent, confidentiality, truth telling, and good communication. More specifically, in cases involving patients who object to a particular medical treatment because of religious or moral considerations, the principle of autonomy weighs in favor of the patient's "virtually absolute veto power."[442] Why? "The ultimate right to select among available treatments, and to refuse any treatment, rests with the patient because it is the patient's body, and in turn the patient's life,

---

[440] *Dobson (Litigation Guardian of) v. Dobson*, Supreme Court of Canada, File No. 26152, December 8, 1999: July 9.

[441] Gillon, "Medical Ethics: Four Principles Plus Attention to Scope," 185.

[442] Bartholome, "A Revolution in Understanding: How Ethics Has Transformed Health Care Decision Making," 9.

that bears the principal effects of any treatment instituted."[443]

Legal recognition of the principle

Courts have long recognized the legal concept of the right of a patient to autonomous decision-making. In 1912, one American judge was of the opinion that "no amount of professional skill can justify the substitution of the will of the surgeon for that of his patient."[444] Two years later, in 1914, noted American judge Cardozo set out the ground rules for autonomy in the medical context when he wrote: "Every human being of adult years and sound mind has a right to determine what shall be done with his own body; and a surgeon who performs an operation without his patient's consent, commits an assault for which he is liable in damages."[445]

However, there are few early decisions on the explicit duty of doctors to obtain consent from patients. The reason for this, wrote the Supreme Court of Canada, in 1945, is that "it is common and obvious." Once the patient has been examined by the doctor and informed of his options, then it is the patient, and only the patient, who can decide which treatment he will consent to.[446] It nevertheless became necessary for the court decisions to go a step further and give substance to this clearly established principle by elaborating a mechanism to make it work. They did this by adopting the doctrine of *informed consent* that specifies exactly how a patient may exercise autonomy or self-determination. This notion will be examined later.

For its part, the Province of Quebec, which has a *civil law* legal system,

---

443 Brock, Medical Ethics, 369.

444 *Bennan v. Parsonnet* (1912), 83 *N.J.L.R.* 20 at 26.

445 *Schloendorff v. Society of New York Hospital, supra* note 246 at 125.

446 Some of the older Canadian decisions on the question are: *Slater v. Baker* (1767) 2 Wils. K.B. 359, 95 E.R. 860; 22 Hals. (2nd ed.) at 319; *Marshall v. Curry,* (1933) 3 D.L.R. 60 Can. C.C. 136 (Nova Scotia); *Mulloy v. Hop Sang,* (1935) 1 W.W.R. 714; *Winn v. Alexander and the Soldiers' Memorial Hospital,* (1940) O.W.N. 238; *Murray v. McMurchy,* (1949) 2 D.L.R. 442; *Kenney v. Lockwood Clinic Ltd.,* (1931) 4 D.L.R. 906, O.R. 438; rev. (1932), 1 D.L.R. 507 O.R. 141 (Ontario).

maintained a paternalist approach to doctor-patient relationship. In 1899, a Montreal judge concluded that a doctor could proceed without consent with a major operation in the course of a minor operation, if the procedure was deemed necessary. Several years later, in 1930, a doctor who had removed a patient's ovaries without consent, during an appendectomy, was unsuccessfully sued. The trial judge viewed beneficence as more important than autonomy. He expressed the prevailing view of this epoch when he stated that in similar cases "there is only the honor between the conscience of the doctor and the patient and between them there is only God as judge."[447] The principles of beneficence and sanctity of life were carried to their limits. This led to the elaboration of the doctrine of 'forced intervention in cases of 'necessity,' a doctrine that was endorsed by leading jurists in the province well into the 1970s.[448] The argument was simple: to be autonomous, one needed to be alive; thus to prevent a doctor from saving someone's life, even against that person's will, violated that same person's autonomy. "Le respect de la vie, parce qu'il est conforme 'a l'intérêt de l'individu,' prime le respect de la volonté" argued Justice Mayrand.[449] Whenever it seemed that a human life was in danger, the doctrine could be applied. Thus, in 1984, Justice Réjean Paul did not hesitate to issue an *ex-parte* order forcing a blood transfusion on a 20-year-old woman suffering from a *post partum* hemorrhage. The argument that her 'life was in danger' seemed to have been unjustified, for upon being advised of the court order, she promptly left the

---

447 *Caron v. Gagnon*, (1930) R.J. at 155. (S. Ct.). According to the trial judge: "Suivant le langage des auteurs, dans les cas graves d'interventions chirurgicales, il n'y a que l'honneur entre la conscience du médecin et le patient, et il n'y a entre eux, pour juge, que Dieu. Le médecin qui a agi d'après son savoir, sa conscience et l'honneur, a bien fait. Toute autre doctrine est fausse et dangereuse à la société."

448 An influential essay on this doctrine was written by Mayrand, L'inviolabilité de la personne humaine, 48-9. The doctrine was adopted in *Boyer v. Grignon*, [1988] R.J.Q. at 829. It was however, severely criticized in Kouri, "Blood Transfusions, Jehovah's Witnesses and the Rule of the Inviolability of the Human Body," 156.

449 Mayrand, L'inviolabilité de la personne humaine, *supra* note 448, 48.

hospital and went to a different one where she was successfully treated according to her wishes.[450] Such abuses led to the demise of the doctrine of 'forced intervention in cases of necessity'. By the end of the 1980s, it had largely been discarded.

Surprisingly, in the Province of Quebec, the principle of autonomy had already been codified into the *Quebec Charter of Human Rights and Freedoms* in 1975. Yet, with regards to health-care, it was not fully enforced by the courts before the late 1980s.[451] It is now part of the new *Quebec Civil Code* that was adopted in 1994.[452]

More astonishing yet, was the strong resistance within the medical community to the principle of autonomy.

Difficult introduction into medicine

While the principle of autonomy has emerged as a most basic and central principle in modern democratic society, it has met with strong resistance from the medical establishment. This was mainly due to the rampant paternalism that had permeated the profession for centuries. Advances in medicine gave physicians increasing power over death. Preoccupied with the "salvation of mankind from attack by illness," they came "to play a role reserved to ministers of religion." As "authority figure(s) in a white coat," they knew what was best for their patients; there was no need to consult.[453]

---

450 *Lakeshore General Hospital v. Methot-Gaudreault*, S. Ct. Montreal, no. 500-05-008750-844, August 1, 1984.

451 See *Weiss v. Solomon* (1989) R.J.Q. 731 (S. Ct.); *Manoir de la Pointe Bleue (1978) Inc. v. Corbeil* (1992) R.J.Q. 712 (S. Ct.). Also the *Quebec Chart of Human Rights* (L.R.Q. c. C-12) adopted in 1975 provided at section 1 that: "Every human being has a right to life, and to personal security, inviolability and freedom." The previous *Civil Code of Lower Canada* also had a similar provision at article 19: "The human person is inviolable. No one may cause harm to the person of another without his consent or without being authorized by law to do so."

452 The *Civil Code of Quebec*, which was adopted in 1994, has the following provision at article 10: "Every person is inviolable and is entitled to the integrity of his person. Except in cases provided for by law, no one may interfere with his person without his free and enlightened consent."

453 Ramsey, The Patient as a Person, *supra* note 453, 137. Ramsey uses this expression when he argues in favor of doctors taking into account not only medical issues but also their patient's wishes or desires.

The doctor-patient relationship was an unequal partnership often dominated by paternalism, that is "the intentional overriding of one person's known preferences or actions by another person, where the person who overrides justifies the action by the goal of benefiting or avoiding harm to the person whose will is overridden."[454] Such a violation of autonomy could be overt or concealed. An example of a covert form of paternalism is the physician who withholds critical information from a patient. This was the situation in the *Pittman*[455] case where the doctor, believing it to be in the best interest of the patient, deliberately omitted advising his patient, Mr Pittman, that he had received blood contaminated with HIV. In the meantime, not knowing he was carrying the virus, Mr Pittman infected his wife.

Paternalism has also been described as an "elaborate charade of parentalism." There existed a myth that a patient, in order to heal, had to place himself entirely into the care of the physician. This "was a complex process in which patients – who were scared and sick – often desperately sought out providers who would take care of them and make things all better again". Patients, "like good children, passively obeyed and complied with the orders" of the doctor.[456] The 'doctor knows best' attitude was the only one. So, for example, when Benjamin Rush ordered yellow fever victims to be bled, there was no resistance. Patients, like little children, did as they were told.

The transition to health-care professionals beginning to respect patients' autonomy was not easy. Early efforts to address medical ethics "from the patient's point of view," such as Joseph Fletcher's 1954 book *Morals and*

"Even when he could succeed, a doctor may and sometimes should allow his medical judgment to defer to a patient's estimate of the higher importance of the worth and the relations for which his life was lived."

[454] Beauchamp, Principles of Biomedical Ethics, *supra* note 434, 274.

[455] *Pittman Estate v. Bain*, *supra* note 189.

[456] Bartholome, "A Revolution in Understanding: How Ethics Has Transformed Health Care Decision Making," *supra* note 442, 7

Medicine, did not change the balance of power.[457] Neither did advances in therapeutics tackling "crippling infectious diseases such as polio and tuberculosis" and "chronic diseases such as cancer and heart disease" improve the doctor-patient relationship. In fact, in the early 1970s it could be said that "medicine was doing better but patients were feeling worse."[458] However, the 'rights' movement of the 1960s was slowly gaining momentum as people insisted on their right as individuals to self-determination in all walks of life. This spilled over into the medical field where government action and court decisions would eventually deal a deathblow to medical paternalism as it had existed for centuries. It became evident that "no man is good enough to cure another without his consent."[459] Today, few health-care professionals advocate outright paternalism; when they do, they find little support and when they act upon it, they often find themselves facing a lawsuit.[460]

Today, only a feeble shadow of past paternalism still lingers among health-care professionals. For example, some authors refer to the overriding of "a *nonautonomous* person's wishes, choices, or actions" who has "compromised ability" as "soft or weak" paternalism.[461] This, however, can hardly be called paternalism, as there is little debate that "persons deserve to be protected from harm caused *to* an individual by conditions *beyond* his or her self-control."[462]

More insidious is "strong or hard" paternalism which is defined as

---

[457] Flecher, Morals and Medicine.

[458] Rothman, Strangers at the Bedside, *supra* note 363 of chapter 5, 107.

[459] Ramsey, The Patient as a Person, *supra* note 453, 7.

[460] See for example *Pittman Estate v. Bain, supra* note 189. In this case the treating physician decided that his patient Mr Pittman "was too emotionally fragile to be told of his transfusion of bad blood." In *Malette v. Shulman, supra* note 269 the treating physician was charged with battery for ignoring the wishes of Mrs Malette expressed in advanced directives and confirmed by her daughter. See also D. Ridley, "Honoring Jehovah's Witnesses' Advance Directives in Emergencies: A Response to Drs Migden and Braen," *supra* note 330 of chapter 4, 833. Author refers to American cases where doctors have been sued for disregarding the wishes of conscientious objectors to blood transfusion.

[461] Childress, *Medical Ethics, supra* note 407, 43.

[462] Beauchamp, Principles of Biomedical Ethics, *supra* note 434 of chapter 5, 277-8.

overriding "an autonomous person's wishes, choices, or actions."[463] Advocates of this approach will argue that such an intervention is intended to benefit the patient where risky choices have been made.[464] In the name of *beneficence*, the physician will justify his action by stating that he has a duty to preserve the life of his patient and to provide appropriate treatments. Or, from a *nonmaleficence* standpoint, he may argue that all unnecessary risks must be avoided in order to avoid harming his patient. Such justification for violating a patient's autonomy does not attract the sympathy of today's courts.

Most physicians have now moved so far away from the extreme paternalistic approach of bygone years that some complain they have gone too far. They want to recapture the lost power for the physician. One writer complains: "Too often, 'autonomous' patients and families are asked to make critical medical decisions on the basis of neutrally presented statistics, as free as possible from the contaminating influences of physicians." Claiming this represents a threat as serious as medical paternalism, he suggests allowing the "physician to support and *guide* the patient's decision making without surrendering the medical power" and would include "strong recommendations and vigorous exchange of ideas and perspective."[465] This approach has the semblance of paternalism. In view of the difficulty of purging long held tenets, vigilance is necessary to avoid the slippery slope of paternalism. While some patients may require *and request* ongoing guidance from the physician for medical decision making, this will not be the case for someone who firmly objects to certain medical treatment on moral or religious grounds. One can easily imagine the harassment of a patient objecting to blood transfusions for religious reasons where the physician has strong personal and

---

463 Childress, *Medical Ethics*, *supra* note 407, 43.

464 Beauchamp, Principles of Biomedical Ethics, *supra* note 434 of chapter 5, 277.

465 Quill, "Physician Recommendations and Patient Autonomy: Finding a Balance between Physician and Patient Choice," 764. The author does admit that there is a "potential for abuse of physician power" under his proposed "relationship-centered model" model.

anti-religious views regarding the objection and insists on *guiding* the patient to make the decision considered medically sound. This issue will be addressed later.

Some form of paternalism may be acceptable and even necessary in some circumstances, such as making choices for those who have never been competent or for those who, once competent, are now incompetent and their prior wishes are unknown or impossible to determine. However, paternalism that violates the autonomy or right to self-determination of a patient cannot be acceptable. As stated by H. Engelhardt, "paternalistic medicine, … may be not only oppressive and vexatious, but in the long run injurious to the health of patients by not encouraging patient responsibility."[466] A paternalistic approach to medicine that is in direct conflict with the autonomy or the right to self-determination of a patient had to be reviewed and eventually discarded.

However, because of the "temptation in medicine to use the authority of the physician's role to foster or perpetuate the dependency of patients", more was needed than simply a principle.[467] Nothing less than a concrete rule that would become both legally and morally binding would suffice. Rising from the ashes of cruel and deadly medical research, the Nuremberg Code made a first attempt by stating: "*The voluntary consent of the human subject is absolutely essential.*" From this evolved the doctrine of 'informed consent,' a concept that would revolutionize the doctor-patient relationship.

---

466 Engelhardt, The Foundations of Bioethics, 320. Englehardt goes on to explain "given particular value commitments, paternalism should not be avoided. One must treat infants in a paternalistic fashion. The very senile must be similarly treated. The moral issue is the extent to which paternalism in health care is allowable and desirable."

467 Beauchamp, Principles of Biomedical Ethics, *supra* note 434 of chapter 5, 127.

8. The Rule of Informed Consent

Physicians today must obtain an informed consent from their patient before proceeding with treatment. It is more than a legal rule that carries grave consequences if violated. It is also an ethical or moral duty imposed on all health-care professionals. Although now considered an essential part of 'good medical care', informed consent is a relatively modern phenomenon.[468] The progress of medicine into the 20th century bestowed upon the physician an unusual power over death.[469] Informed consent evolved as a needed response, as a counterbalance, with a view to protecting patients.

Development of the principle and its application

The need to obtain consent from patients was made disturbingly evident during the Nuremberg trials. "University trained and university appointed researchers" who "possessed first rate medical credentials and had pursued notable careers" had carried out merciless experimentation on helpless victims during the Nazi regime.[470] Humans were tortured and murdered to serve the goals of science and medicine. The medicine man, without rules or laws, had run amok. One author catalogued some of the terrible atrocities committed: "Among the studies in which human beings were used in research were the analysis of high-

---

468 Nora, "Medicolegal Aspects of Informed Consent," 214.

469 Illich, Limits to Medicine, 205. The author, commenting on the power of physicians over death, writes: "Like all other major rituals of industrial society, medicine in practice takes the form of a game. The chief function of the physician becomes that of an umpire. He is the agent or representative of the social body, with the duty to make sure that everyone plays the game according to the rules. The rules, of course, forbid leaving the game and dying in any fashion that has not been specified by the umpire. Death no longer occurs except as the self-fulfilling prophecy of the medicine man."

470 Rothman, Strangers at the Bedside, *supra* note 363 of chapter 5, 63.

altitude decompression on the human body; attempts to make sea water drinkable; the efficacy of sulfanilamide for treating gunshot wounds; the feasibility of bone, muscle, and joint transplants; the ability to treat burns caused by incendiary bombs; the efficacy of polygal for treating trauma-related bleeding; the efficacy of high-dose radiation in causing sterility; the efficacy of phenol (gasoline) injections as a euthanasia agent; the efficacy of electroshock therapy; the symptoms and course of noma (starvation-caused skin gangrene); the postmortem examination of skeletons and brains to assess the effects of starvation; the efficacy of surgical techniques for sterilizing women; and the impact of stress and starvation on ovulation, menstruation, and cancerous growths in the reproductive organs of women. A variety of other studies were carried out on twins, dwarves, and those with congenital defects. Some camp inmates were used as subjects to train medical students in surgery."[471]

The "bedrock principle of medical ethics – that the physician acted only to promote the well-being of the patient" had been grossly violated.[472] The Nuremberg trials resulted in the Nuremberg Code that sought to prevent a repetition of atrocities such as those perpetrated by physicians under the Nazi regime, by imposing the duty of obtaining voluntary consent from research subjects. This new requirement did not, however, result in any major changes in the patient-doctor relationship. In fact, in the United States, experimentation without consent from the patient continued well into the late 1960s.

In 1965, a researcher, by the name of H. Beeker, upset some of his colleagues during a lecture in which he presented evidence that dangerous medical experimentation was being carried out on unwitting patients in the United States.

---

[471] Enlow, "The German Medical War Crimes: Their Nature and Significance," 801-5. See also Lifton, The Nazi Doctor: Medical Killing and the Psychology of Genocide; Capland, When Medicine Went Mad: Bioethics and the Holocaust, 64; See also Annas, The Nazi Doctors and the Nuremberg Code; Ivy, "Nazi War Crimes of a Medical Nature," 131; Alexander, "Medical Science Under Dictatorship," 39.

[472] Rothman, Strangers at the Bedside, *supra* note 363 of chapter 5, 89.

They accused him of being an "irresponsible exaggerator."[473] Undaunted, he went on to publish the information in a medical journal in 1966.[474] In this article, which received extensive media attention, he submitted 22 examples of published studies carried out by American researchers in which the health and safety of patients were endangered without their knowledge. Among the "troubling practices" engaged in without the consent or knowledge of patients and documented by Beecher were: injection of live cancer cells in human subjects; induction of hepatitis in mentally defective children; insertion of a needle through a bronchus into the left atrium of the heart; exploration of physiologic responses and testing of new drugs. Seemingly unperturbed by the lack of informed consent, prominent university medical school clinics such as Harvard Medical School and Georgetown University, along with leading professors and investigators, were involved in these questionable studies.[475]

This revelation led to legal and ethical debates that eventually resulted in the establishing of an obligation in both research and clinical settings to obtain consent from adequately informed patients before proceeding with any medical intervention.

Informed consent is now mandatory. It has been defined as "an *autonomous authorization* by individuals of a medical intervention or of involvement in research." Such an authorization needs to meet both ethical principles and legal rules. From an ethical viewpoint, the notions of informed consent have been described as follows:

I. Threshold Elements (Preconditions)

1. Competence (to understand and decide)
2. Voluntariness (in deciding)

II. Information Elements

---

473 *Ibid.*, 72.

474 Bleecher, "Ethics and Clinical Research," 1354.

475 Rothman, Strangers at the Bedside, *supra* note 363 of chapter 5, 77-8.

3. Disclosure (of material information)
4. Recommendation (of a plan)
5. Understanding (of 3. and 4.)

III. Consent Elements

6. Decision (in favor of a plan)
7. Authorization (of a chosen plan)[476]

As one writer noted, "a review of informed consent leaves one with a sense that medical standards and ethical standards on this issue are more stringent than the legal ones."[477] Naturally, whatever the standard used, the elements of informed consent must be such that the average person will be able to make autonomous choices without having to meet such high standards that only a few educated and reflective individuals could qualify to make medical choices.

While the extent to which the above-mentioned elements of informed consent are fully implemented may vary from one physician to another, they will, nevertheless, all need to meet minimal *legal* requirements. The Canadian Supreme Court in the *Hopp v. Lepp* case described this minimal threshold as follows: In summary, the decided cases appear to indicate that, in obtaining the consent of a patient for the performance upon him of a surgical operation, a surgeon, generally, *should answer* any specific questions posed by the patient as to the risks involved and should, without being questioned, *disclose* to him the nature of the proposed operation, its gravity, any material risks and any *special or unusual risks* attendant upon the performance of the operation.[478] [emphasis added]

The *Hopp v. Lepp* case, described as "strong medicine to improve the

---

476 Beauchamp, Principles of Biomedical Ethics, *supra* note 434 of chapter 5, 145-6. For a discussion of each element see pp 146-170.

477 Nora, "Medicolegal Aspects of Informed Consent," *supra* note 468, 214 .

478 *Hopp v. Lepp*, [1980] 2 S.C.R. 192 at 210. See also companion case *Reibl v. Hughes*, [1980] 2 S.C.R. 180 at 184.

doctor-patient relationship," established the standard of full disclosure by the doctor (of information pertinent to the particular patient) before obtaining consent, failing which a negligence action could ensue.[479] As a result, physicians are encouraged to maintain "good patient communication" and to make use of "education materials, including written forms, videotapes, or other documents" to educate their patient about the proposed intervention.[480] Consent should never be "taken for granted."[481]

Even though today consent is a well established legal and ethical requirement, in general it has not been applied to the administration of blood or blood products. For example, the Canadian Krever Commission, which investigated the tainted blood scandal in the mid-90s, observed that it was not the general practice of Canadian hospitals to obtain informed consent before administering blood transfusion. The Commission was however, of the opinion that informed consent should be obtained. In his *Interim Report*, Justice Krever wrote: "There is a growing realization that patients who may be given a transfusion of allogeneic blood (blood from one or more other persons) in the course of treatment should be advised of the risks and benefits involved, and of the alternatives open to them. ... There is a growing sense that the treating physician should obtain the patient's prior consent to any administration of blood and blood products."[482]

---

479 Picard "Consent to Medical Treatment in Canada," 140. The basic requirement of disclosure was "what the average prudent person, the reasonable person in the patient's particular position, would agree to or not agree to, if all material and special risks of going ahead with the surgery or foregoing it were made known to him." See Rozovsky, The Canadian Law of Consent to Treatment, 8.

480 Nora, "Medicolegal Aspects of Informed Consent," *supra* note 468, 214. See also Loyd, "Patients' Ability to Recall Risk Associated With Treatment Options," 645 and response by Gattellari., "Informed Consent: What Did the Doctor Say?" 1713. (Discussion of patient's understanding and remembering information given to them by the physician and the use of information aids.)

481 Horty, "Informed Consent: Patient Can Set Limits," 16.

482 Krever, Commission of Inquiry on the Blood System in Canada, *supra* note 3 of the Introduction, 61. See also Capen, "Informed Consent and Blood Transfusions: What Does Krever's Interim Report Mean to Doctors?" 1663. In this article, the author highlights the importance of good communication between the physician and the patient on the issue of blood transfusion in order to obtain true consent instead of relying solely on a written consent form." During July, 1999, inquiries were made by Anne-

Some physicians argue that it is impossible to obtain a truly informed consent – as it would involve communicating to the patient a physician's understanding of the "goals, nature and hazards" of the proposed procedure.[483] Adopting such a view would mean that only doctors and well educated individuals could truly exercise the right of self-determination in a medical setting. All others would be obliged to defer to the physician, resulting in a gross violation of the principle of autonomy. A more reasonable approach recognizes the positive right of consent of individuals, a right that flows from their very status as persons.

Given sufficient information relative to the purpose at hand, competent patients can, and do, make "meaningful decisions" that permit them to give truly 'informed consent.'[484] So, the *competence* of the individual must be considered when obtaining informed consent, explicit or implicit. As mentioned by justice Cardozo "(e)very human being of adult years and *sound mind* has a right to determine what shall be done with his own body."[485] Adults are presumed competent and it is those who claim incompetence who must "bear the onus of supporting their assertion."[486] While there are many theories on competency, "competence is determined primarily by whether a person has the capacity to decide autonomously, and not by whether a person's best interests are

---

Marie Gaucher, MD with 15 Montreal area hospital regarding obtaining specific consent for blood transfusion. Nine hospitals respond. Of the nine, only one hospital was using a specific consent form for all blood transfusions. In the other eight cases, consent was obtained only for prolonged programs of blood transfusion. In the United States, the Joint Commission on Accreditation of Healthcare Organizations has specifically required that institutions document informed consent for transfusion. See Sazama, "Practical Issues in Informed Consent for Transfusion," S72.

483 Ingelfinger, "Informed (But Uneducated) Consent," 465.

484 Freedman, "A Moral Theory of Consent," 5. See also Grisso, Evaluating Competencies – Forensic Assessments and Instruments, 320. "The abilities in question are not a patient's aptitude for reasoning about information concerning the world in general, but rather the capacity to reason with information of a type relevant for treatment decisions."

485 See *supra* note 246.

486 Madigan, "Presumptions Respecting Mental Competence," 147.

protected."[487]

Consent and refusal treated differently

While this has not always been the case, today there is general agreement that "(t)he right to consent comprehends the right to refuse."[488] If the patient decides to refuse a particular treatment when exercising his right of informed consent (refusal), the physician is then "stripped of professional authority and power and is left to plead with the patient and to use the only force any of us should have over the lives of others, namely that of language or moral persuasion."[489]

Some physicians, however, have difficulty accepting that their patient may not always agree with proposed treatment. In fact, if a patient refuses a recommended treatment, his competency may well be questioned and an assessment of competency requested, "often with the clear expectation that the patient will be found incompetent so that treatment can proceed."[490] However, it has been noted that the majority of patients refusing treatment are found to be competent.[491] Therefore, sensible measures taken to assist a patient understand the consequences of a particular choice need not degenerate into paternalism, whereby patients' competence is unquestioned as long as they concur with the doctor.

---

[487] Beauchamp, Principles of Biomedical Ethics, *supra* note 434 of chapter 5, 141. Some have proposed a sliding-scale strategy in which competency is directly related to the risk attached to the decision. See Drane, "Competency to Give an informed Consent: A Model for Making Clinical Assessments." Others have proposed different standards of abilities or skills to assess competence such as ability to state a preference, abilities to understand information and to appreciate one's situation and ability to reason through a consequential life decision. See Beauchamp, Principles of Biomedical Ethics, *supra* note 434 of chapter 5, 136-8.

[488] Emson, The Doctor and the Law, 126.

[489] Bartholome, "A Revolution in Understanding: How Ethics Has Transformed Health Care Decision Making," *supra* note 442, 9.

[490] Katz, "Psychiatric Consultation for Competency to Refuse Medical Treatment," 34.

[491] *Ibid.*

If the principles of autonomy and self-determination are to be respected, the right to consent means the right to make a choice. The choice of accepting or refusing proposed treatment belongs to the patient, and the patient alone. Medically, the physician may not agree with the decision, but must finally defer to the reality that all ethical principles and rules need give way to the "fundamental right" of patients to determine what shall be done to their body. "The concepts inherent in this right are the bedrock upon which the principles of self-determination and individual autonomy are based."[492] While this seems to be an established fundamental rule in the practice of modern medicine, physicians nevertheless are recurrently reminded that "the code of ethics of our profession clearly recognizes a patient's right to reject any medical care recommended."[493]

Informed consent in emergency situations through advanced directives

There is however, an exception to the rule of informed consent. This is when the physician proceeds in an emergency situation where the patient is in life- or health-threatening circumstances and is unable to give consent. In these urgent circumstances, the physician may proceed with "treatment that is necessary for the sake of the life or health of the patient"[494] if, according to the College of Physicians and Surgeons of Ontario, the following criteria are met:

1. The patient must be unconscious or incapable of making a decision, and without the presence of someone who is legally competent to make the decision.
2. The patient must need treatment immediately to preserve health or prevent death.

---

[492] *Malette v.Shulman, supra* note 269 at 336.

[493] Overs, "Patients can refuse treatment by MD," 8.

[494] Rozovsky, The Canadian Law of Consent to Treatment, 20; See also *Marshall v. Curry, supra* 446; *Murray v. McMurchy, supra* 446; *Parmley v. Parmley* [1945] 4 D.L.R. 81 (S.C.C.).

3. A reasonable person would consent to the treatment, and it is probable that this patient would consent if conscious and capable of giving or withholding consent.[495]

When these conditions are met, and medical treatment is provided without consent, one cannot say that the patient's autonomy has been violated. In the absence of the ability to exercise one's right to self-determination, the principles of beneficence and nonmaleficence will prevail. However, the emergency treatment doctrine applies only if "under the circumstances, a reasonable person would consent and the probabilities are the patient would consent."[496] If there are clear indications, such as a living will, that the patient would not consent to the proposed treatment, then even in an emergency situation, the physician cannot proceed.

This principle is clearly set out in the *Quebec Civil Code* at article 13 where "consent to medical care is not required in the case of emergency" unless "the care is unusual or has become useless or where its consequences could be intolerable for the person."[497]

However, if a physician is to know that certain 'care' or treatment is unacceptable or intolerable to a patient, some form of advance directives will be necessary, preferably in writing. Many individuals have opted for this. In 1992, for example, it was estimated thousands of living will forms had been distributed across Canada and more that 10 million advanced directives (living wills) had been executed in the United States.[498]

---

495 *College Notices*, Issue No. 21 (November 1990) put out by The College of Physicians and Surgeons of Ontario.

496 Proposals for an Advance Health Care Directive Act, Law Reform Commission of Saskatchewan, Report to the Minister of Justice (December 1991) 11.

497 Article 13 of the *Quebec Civil Code* reads: "Consent to medical care is not required in case of emergency if the life of the person is in danger or his integrity is threatened and his consent cannot be obtained in due time. It is required, however, where the care is unusual or has become useless or where its consequences could be intolerable for the person."

498 Downie, "Where There is a Will, The May Be a Better Way: Legislating Advanced Directives," 73. On early attempts by Canadian provinces to introduce living wills legislation see Linden, "Living Wills

In Canada, in what was probably the first decision to recognize "a specific form of written advance directive for medical treatment" the issue of consent through advanced directives was thoroughly canvassed by the Ontario courts in the *Malette v. Shulman* case.[499] It is noteworthy in that the Canadian Medical Practitioners Association viewed the decision as both legally and morally correct. President Normand Belliveau stated: "The law is quite clear on this and we couldn't find any error in law in the judgment, so we had no real basis for appeal. If we feel we have a leg to stand on, we'll go all the way to the Supreme Court of Canada to defend our doctors but in this case, we just didn't have that leg to stand on, neither in conscience nor in law."[500]

In this case, the Advance Medical Directive carried by Jehovah's Witnesses, requesting that alternatives to blood or blood products be used even in a life-threatening situation, was found to be a valid expression of a person's wishes regarding medical treatment. A physician disregarding it, even in an attempt to save the patient's life, is liable in battery.[501]

In the *Malette* case, the treating physician had disregarded the "unqualified instructions" set out in Mrs Malette's *Advance Medical Directive* card and as a result he was charged with battery. In this unfortunate situation, described as a "continuing battle between a patient's rights and a physician's obligations" the

---

and Substitute Decision-Making," 33.

499 *Malette v. Shulman, supra* note 269 and accompanying text. See also Wahi, "Are Living Wills Valid?" 38. Author comments that the *Malette* decision is the "first in Canada to recognize a specific form of written advance directive for medical treatment."

500 Trent, "Jehovah's Witnesses and the Transfusion Debate: "We Are Not Asking for the Right to Die," 774.

501 See Rozovsky, "Jehovah's Witness Case Sets Precedent – Controversy Over a Patient's Right to Refuse Treatment," 68. According to the author "This decision makes it clear that any doctor giving a blood transfusion to an unconscious patient in contravention of a written notification not to do so, will be liable in battery, even though the result may be to save the life of the patient." This author who is an important contributor to medicolegal writings had earlier that the Advance Medical Directive was invalid because the patient had signed it when not confronted with the emergency. The *Malette* decision corrected this erroneous viewpoint. See Rozovsky, Canadian Hospital Law, 39-40.

victory was clearly on the side of respect for patients' autonomy.[502] Be it in respect to advance directives or a contemporaneous expression of one's wishes, a greater significance will be placed on a patient's values and preferences than on the physician's values and obligations. In light of modern medical ethics, this is the correct approach, since, as Ramsey expressed it, "no man is good enough to cure another without his consent."[503]

---

502 Rozovsky, "Jehovah's Witness Case Sets Precedent – Controversy Over a Patient's Right to Refuse Treatment," *supra* note, 501, 68.

503 Ramsey, The Patient as a Person, *supra* note 436 of chapter 7.

9. When Traditional Rules are Not Enough

The greatest dangers to liberty lurk in insidious encroachment by men of zeal, well-meaning, but without understanding.

Justice L. Brandeis[504]

"One of the more challenging ethical and medicolegal issues that many physicians face is caring for the patient who refuses specific therapeutic interventions based on religious or social dogma."[505] To address this issue and endeavor to determine the rules or principles that apply, the example of Jehovah's Witnesses has been chosen. Given their longstanding conscientious objection to blood transfusion and the dilemma it has posed for physicians, they "provide the largest single group of patients with a clearly defined belief, totally at odds with one type of potentially life saving medical treatment."[506] Ethical and legal solutions found to be successful in managing their situation, without violating their dignity and autonomy, could possibly find application to the circumstances of other conscientious objectors.

When confronted with a patient who refuses blood transfusion because of religious beliefs, many physicians seem perplexed; "confusion" and even "emotional bias" often set in.[507] In this context of religious and moral disagreement, where "(t)he occupational hazard of medicine is arrogance," some patients have been "clandestinely transfused … or abandoned to truly suboptimal management, making death inevitable."[508] On the issue of abandoning a patient

---

[504] *Olmstead v. US*, 277 US 472 at 479 (1927) Justice Brandeis.

[505] Rothenberg, "The Approach to the Jehovah's Witness Patient," 589.

[506] Gilmartin, Ethical issues in Anesthesia, *supra* note 379 of chapter 6, 106.

[507] *Supra* note 373 and accompanying text.

[508] Elliot, "Second Opinions: A Right or a Concession?" 671; Henry, "Emergency Treatment of Jehovah's Witnesses," 626; See also Ferdinand, "Jehovah's Witnesses and Advance Directives," 64 for

because of his refusal of blood transfusions, author Spence writes: "(T)his has led to past disasters, with Jehovah's Witness patients bleeding to death from surgically correctable lesions while physicians have stood by. We have received many transfer patients in shock, having extremely low Hb levels, who subsequently died. Many could have been saved if earlier action had been taken."[509]

Not only does treating patients in this manner fall far below an acceptable standard of care, it is immoral, unethical, and illegal.

To insist on a therapy that entails potentially lethal risks and has been refused by the patient, might arguably be attributed to what has been called "blind adherence to a therapeutic regimen."[510] After all, a 'mystical aura' has been attached to the use of blood throughout history and blood's 'reputation of mythical proportions' and its 'magical' properties have made it a favorite amongst doctors for millenniums, and continues to be so today.[511]

Interestingly, the 'mystical aura' continued as euphoria over the use of blood as the 'gift of life' gained momentum. During the past century, practices revolving around transfusion medicine developed into "long-held dogmas" difficult to modify.[512] "Over-enthusiastic transfusionists" with a "shallow and narrow understanding" of blood medicine transfused needlessly, causing the death of many.[513] Unnecessary transfusions were often the result of an "excessive and

---

[509] Spence, "The Status of Bloodless Surgery," 284.

[510] *Supra* note 131 and accompanying text.

[511] *Supra* note 199 and accompanying text.

[512] Henry, "Emergency Treatment of Jehovah's Witnesses," *supra* note 508, 627.

[513] *Supra* notes 188 & 198 and accompanying text. When testifying before the Krever Commission, victims of AIDS through contaminated blood administered to them without their consent seriously questioned "whether a blood transfusion was medically indicated." See H. Krever, "Interim Report" in *Commission of Inquiry on the Blood System in Canada, supra* note 3, 62-3. See also S. Saxena, "Iron-Deficiency Anemia: A Medically Treatable Chronic Anemia as a Model for Transfusion Overuse" (1993) 94 Amerc. J. Of Med. 121.

unfounded fear of the risk from not transfusing."[514] Then, the full reality of the lethal dangers of blood therapy became disturbingly evident as tens of thousands in different parts of the world received blood contaminated with HIV and hepatitis.

Even after clear evidence of the serious dangers associated with blood medicine was made public during the blood scandal years, individuals continued to be pressured into consenting to the treatment. One man, C. Labelle, went to Montreal's Sacré-Coeur Hospital on 5 November 1991 for heart bypass surgery. After the surgery, he remained anemic and lethargic. The doctors recommended a blood transfusion to get him back on his feet, but Labelle had heard, through the media, about the tainted blood problem and refused to consent. The attending nurse was sent in to explain and convince him that 'It is impossible to get AIDS from blood since all blood is tested'. Mr Labelle acquiesced and by November 1993 he was dead from AIDS. As he had feared, the blood was contaminated.[515]

The 'magic' of blood transfusions is slowly fading; somewhat mimicking the fate of bloodletting. Physicians are being made aware of the legal ramifications of blindly administering blood.[516] Bloodless surgery is rapidly becoming prominent.[517] Some even predict that it "is quite possible in the very near future [blood] transfusion will be eliminated altogether."[518]

While many in the medical community still view blood as 'life saving,'[519]

---

514 Kitchens, "Are Transfusions Overrated? Surgical Outcome of Jehovah's Witnesses," *supra* note 334,

515 See Picard, The Gift of Death, *supra* note 167 of chapter 2, 225.

516 Clay, "Ethical and Legal Implications of Bloodless Medicine and Surgery," 34, 37; Burns, "When Patients Refuse Blood Transfusion: Meeting the Medical and Legal Challenge," 261.

517 See *supra* Chapter 1, section C, number 3. Medical Alternatives to Blood Transfusion.

518 Godec, chairman of urology at Long Island College Hospital, in Brooklyn, New York, quoted in "Are Blood Transfusions Really Necessary?" Awake!, 31. See also Kreidie, "Bloodless Surgery Making a Comeback with Patients," 21.

519 The Royal College of Surgeons of England, Code of Practice for the Surgical Management of Jehovah's Witnesses, *supra* 338, 1 states: "Nevertheless, a number of conditions can only be successfully treated by homologous transfusion. These include some anaemias and excessive blood loss."

alternate forms of treatment are proving to be 'life saving.'[520] As expressed by E. Rosam, spokesman for Jehovah's Witnesses and longtime liaison agent with the medical community: "The fact is that the vast majority of Jehovah's Witnesses who refuse 'life-saving' blood transfusions do not die. So, if they refuse a 'life-saving' blood transfusion and yet do not die, then the treatment that they did accept must also be 'life-saving.'"[521]

It is becoming evident, contrary to popular belief, that refusing a blood transfusion is not medically irrational and does not automatically lead to death.[522]

Witnesses have had to fight strenuously for their right to refuse what they believe to be a religiously unacceptable medical treatment. This has been done in part through the courts. However, they have also endeavored to educate the medical community on both their religious stance and on the viability of alternatives to blood transfusion. At the same time their Hospital Liaison Committees have successfully promoted and advocated a better doctor-patient relationship. As a result, many physicians, experienced in treating Jehovah's Witnesses, now have an improved understanding of the ability of the body to heal

---

[520] Spence, "Transfusion and Surgery," *supra* note 74, 1109. See also *supra* notes 297-318 and accompanying text.

[521] Rosam, "Patients' Rights and the Role of the Emergency Physician in the Management of Jehovah's Witnesses," *supra* note 337, 1150. See also Kitchens, "Are Transfusions Overrated? Surgical Outcome of Jehovah's Witnesses," *supra* note 334, 119: "Are the benefits of transfusion greatly overrated? If not transfusing Jehovah's Witnesses actually results in little acute extra morbidity and mortality and avoids a significant amount of costs and chronic complications, should patients receive fewer transfusions? Indeed, authors of these very reports have raised this question and have extended these practices (i.e., fewer or no transfusions and the use of normovolemic hemodilution and hypotensive anesthesia) to their routine patients."

[522] See *supra* Chapter 1, section C, number 3. Medical Alternatives to Blood Transfusion. It is now becoming more and more common to hear reports of complicated surgery being performed without the use of blood. For example, on 25 June 1999 DateLine NBC aired a program entitled "Keeping the Faith: Bloodless Surgery." NBC's chief science correspondent, Robert Bazell, reported on 18 year old Stacey Singletary's successful brain surgery. Dr Frank Forte of Englewood Hospital, New Jersey, performed the complicated surgery, without the use of blood transfusion. Another example, was on 4 February 1999, a Montreal daily reported that an open-heart operation had been successfully performed on a two-year-old infant without blood transfusion. See Duma, "Bambin opéré sans transfusion sanguine," A14.

without the use of transfused blood.[523] There is a growing consensus that bloodless medicine makes good sense and many have implemented such programs in their hospitals.[524]

The gradual success of the Witnesses in having their stance respected by health-care professionals reveals that it is possible for physicians to resolve the issue posed by patients who refuse a particular medical treatment for religious or moral reasons. However, to meet that challenge, physicians must look beyond the traditional rules of 'informed consent.' While these rules are adequate for most patients, other guidelines are needed when a patient has determined beforehand that a particular medical treatment violates a deeply held belief. In these cases, the need to be informed must necessarily switch from the patient to the doctor, as the information required is outside the realm of medicine.

In fact, when there is a religiously or morally motivated refusal of a recommended medical treatment, an "informed doctor" is the key to avoiding confrontation. As stated by one author "whether or not a physician supports the Witnesses' beliefs, all physicians must understand their patient's religious credos concerning medicine."[525] The physician, in harmony with the patient's wishes and beliefs, needs to make 'intelligent informed choices' as to how to treat the patient, which alternatives to recommend or, if necessary, where to transfer the patient.

In matters of moral or religious disagreement, ignorance can breed intolerance, and intolerance on the part of a physician can be deadly for the patient. However, an 'informed doctor' will be more likely to treat the "patient as a person" and not simply as a "customer" or a "case."[526]

---

[523] *Supra* note 316 and accompanying text.

[524] *Supra* notes 296-322 and accompanying text.

[525] Findley & Fletcher, "Jehovah's Witnesses and the Right to Refuse Blood," 64.

[526] Argy, "Standards of Care," 1296.

Traditional rules of informed consent are insufficient

Informed consent is the gateway to a patient's autonomy.[527] The patient is the one who decides which treatment to accept, if any. The decision of the patient "will be based on information given by the clinician." While consent forms may be signed, these in reality only "document that some discussion has taken place." It is during these discussions, that the physician is expected to provide information "in a manner intelligible to the hearer and at a pace at which the recipient can digest it." This information must include available alternatives and associated risks. The patient will then exercise his autonomy "by deciding which treatment option to accept."[528]

This approach addresses the issue of consent from the 'patient needs to know' viewpoint and protects the patient from unwanted or unsolicited medical intervention. The physician has the ethical and legal responsibility to provide medical information to a patient and should be "caringly available" to assist in clarifying "any misconceptions."[529] Applying the informed consent rules will result in a patient knowing of, and understanding, available options as well as their risks and benefits. The patient's final decision should thus be an enlightened one, one with which the physician can usually agree.

However, in resolving religious or moral objections to a particular therapy, medical information is not the most important factor. Since the decision of the patient is not premised on medical information alone but also on religious or moral belief, putting undue emphasis on transmitting medical information and trying to convince the patient to accept an objectionable treatment may in fact result in a breakdown of communication and be detrimental to the care of the patient. The individual's values, beliefs and wishes must take precedence over the

---

[527] See *supra* Chapter 2, Section C: The Rule of Informed Consent.

[528] Sommerville, Medical Ethics Today: Its Practice and Philosophy, 7-9.

[529] *Ibid.*, 8.

physician's values, beliefs and wishes.

When medical information becomes of secondary importance

The secondary importance of medical information regarding a proposed treatment which has been refused for religious or moral reasons becomes evident in the case of Jehovah's Witnesses who "have *absolutely* refused the transfusion of blood and primary blood components ever since these techniques became universally available. Theirs is a *deeply-held* core value."[530] Their position is "*non-negotiable*."[531] Since, from the outset, treatment with blood is unacceptable, information regarding such treatment would hardly be of primary importance. The most pressing issue is to understand the religious or moral objection of the patient and to respect it. Following the rules of informed consent, discussion on other possible treatment ensues and acceptable alternatives should be sought and proposed. This would apply not only to Jehovah's Witnesses, but also to others, such as a Roman Catholic who, for religious reasons, absolutely refuses an abortion, or to a Muslim or to a Jew who will not consent to treatment involving pork derivatives.[532]

While the physician should be concerned that the patient understands the possible risks of the alternative treatment and the benefits of the proposed treatment, the deeply held beliefs of the individual must be understood and respected. Only an 'informed doctor' will be adequately prepared to do so.

To focus solely on the medical information regarding a proposed treatment would miss the real objective of the informed consent process. The principle of informed consent was developed to protect the patient's autonomy from the encroachments of medical paternalism. Respect for a patient's deeply held beliefs and values are at the very heart of the autonomy of that person. However, conflict

---

[530] The Royal College of Surgeons of England, Code of Practice for the Surgical Management of Jehovah's Witnesses, *supra* note 338 of chapter 4, 1.

[531] How Can Blood Save Your Life?, *supra* note 5 of chapter 1.

[532] See Manners, "When Religious Faith Dictates Treatment," *supra* note 4 of chapter 1, 17-18.

may seem unavoidable when a patient refuses what is perceived by the physician to be life-saving treatment for religious or moral reasons. After all, the physician's "first and primary goal is to support life." Nevertheless, if the physician switches his focus from the 'informed patient' to the 'informed doctor' approach, there is greater likelihood that the patient's beliefs and values will be properly addressed without undue frustration on the part of the physician.

Need for physicians to be properly informed

One survey revealed that of those who responded, most physicians and medical students did not understand why Jehovah's Witnesses refuse blood. The survey concluded that "professionals need to know more about Witnesses, why they refuse transfusion, and how strongly they believe in the refusal."[533] These poorly informed physicians, when faced with a Witness patient who refuses a blood transfusion, often react with "anger" and "frustration." They may resort to "(t)actics of opposition (which) too often include emotionally loaded persuasion, threats, deception, and withdrawal from the patient's care."[534] Such actions can hardly be considered a proper standard of care.

In contrast, the properly 'informed doctor', armed with an understanding of the beliefs and values of the patient, as well as information on acceptable alternatives, will be empowered to "provide net medical benefit to patients with minimal harm – that is beneficence with non-malfeasance."[535] This, an

---

533 Duh, "Physician Reaction to Refusal of Blood Transfusions by Jehovah's Witnesses," 467.

534 Andrews, "Legal, Ethical, and Medical Guidelines for Jehovah's Witnesses in Surgery," *supra* note 354 of chapter 4, 2.

535 Gillon, "Medical Ethics: Four Principles Plus Attention to Scope," *supra* 441 of chapter 7, 185; Legal advisers are warning physicians to "assess the efficacy and safety of the treatment" before proceeding with blood transfusion therapy. This will involve keeping up to date with information regarding the risks associated to blood as well as new alternatives available. Physicians should obtain the patient's specific consent before administering blood products. See Clay, "Ethical and Legal Implications of Bloodless Medicine and Surgery," *supra* note 516, 37. See also Grainger, "Legal and Ethical Considerations in Blood Transfusion," 550.

appropriate and proper standard of care, will "not only respect but also enhance" the patient's autonomy.[536]

[536] R. Gillon, "Medical Ethics: Four Principles Plus Attention to Scope," *supra* 441, 185.

10. Informed Doctor More Likely to Respect Patient's Beliefs

Transfusion certainly makes the surgeon feel better, but it may not make the patient feel better. Perhaps we all have a tendency to transfuse to make ourselves more comfortable. I think when we have a Jehovah's Witness, we'll do well to consider his point of view.

Dr Englbert Dunphy[301]

When a physician disagrees with a Witness patient who refuses a blood transfusion, often the "root of the controversy lies not in the patient's convictions, which are usually firm, but in the physician's inability to accept the stipulation and proceed with care."[537] This has been described as the "physician denial of patients' ability to choose rational, ethically sound medical or life goals." Remnant of paternalism, such a denial represents a serious "threat to autonomy and well-being."[538]

Today's physicians are faced with the reality that their "instincts to protect patients against their own decisions, including the conscientious instinct to sustain life, are limited by law."[539] The physician is no longer 'alone with his patient and God.'

Ethical standards, however, transcend basic legal requirements. They are a constantly evolving paradigm of ethical behavior for the physician.[540] Based on the premise that the patient's right to self-determination supercedes the physician's "privilege to treat their patients,"[541] medical practitioners are encouraged to "explore the reasoning" and "understand the values and goals that

---

537 Cooper "Preoperative Considerations in Jehovah's Witnesses," 210

538 Meyers, "The Impact of Physician Denial Upon Patient Autonomy and Well-Being," 135.

539 Dickens, "Medical Priority of Patient's Wishes," 9.

540 Parizeau & Carbonneau, Consentement éclairé et transfusion sanguine, 161.

541 Thomas, "Ethical Reflections on Patient Refusals of Life-Saving Treatment," 259.

underlie decisions to refuse care."[542] This is particularly important when the refusal is based on religious or moral considerations. As one author observes, such an approach fosters a good relationship: "(T)he patient's perception is influenced by the physician through effective communication, clinical acumen, and empathy. Physicians will enhance their relationships with patients by displaying these skills and concern, and the patient will perceive the reality that the physician is an ally and not an adversary."[543]

For example, if the physician comprehends that with the Witness patient the issue "is not merely the low degree of bodily invasion, but the violation of the integrity of the person as encompassing psychological, social, spiritual, as well as physical, well-being," it will be easier to appreciate that not to respect the patient's refusal of blood therapy would be "a personal insult of a very deep and cutting nature."[544]

Progressive physicians, up-to-date with contemporary medical developments, understand that the request for non-blood management can also be scientifically sound. Clinical alternatives are available, effective, and becoming an accepted part of current medical practice. The dramatic rise of centers for bloodless medicine and surgery shows that concerns about allogeneic blood are no longer of a strictly religious nature.[545] "The recent shift away from the liberal use of transfusions in clinical medicine suggests that the standard of practice regarding the use of allogeneic blood is undergoing significant revision."[546]

---

542 Adams, "Respecting the Right to Be Wrong," *supra* note 267 of chapter 2.

543 See Argy, "Another Standard of Care – Patient, In Reply," 450.

544 Thomas, "Ethical Reflections on Patient Refusals of Life-Saving Treatment," *supra* note 541, 260; Wreen, "Autonomy, Religious Values, and Refusal of Lifesaving Medical Treatment," 128.

545 *Supra* notes 317-319 of chapter 3 an accompanying text.

546 Clay, "Ethical and Legal Implications of Bloodless Medicine and Surgery," *supra* note 516, 37.

Unethical coercion

As stated earlier, some authors have proposed a form of paternalistic intervention in which the physician, having decided what is best for the patient, then proceeds to argue with the objective of changing the patient's views on the issue.[547] Such a coercive, almost "evangelical" approach is clearly unethical in the presence of deeply held values and beliefs. In a reversal of roles, one could hardly imagine the health-care profession tolerating a physician, himself one of Jehovah's Witnesses, attempting to convert patients to the belief that blood transfusions are a grave violation of God's law and must be avoided at all cost! No physician should try to impose personal values and beliefs on a patient. Such attempts are not only unethical but are also counterproductive, "leading to destruction of the doctor-patient relationship."[548]

Also to be considered is the unfair advantage the physician has over the patient in the medical arena. The ailing patient has left his social environment and enters the hospital, "a stranger in a strange land – in a world of which he knows neither the language, the rites nor the traditions."[549] This "patient in pajamas" must now confront the "authority figure in a white coat." Secure in his element, the physician is armed with scientific and medical knowledge, empowered and determined to save lives. Given the setting, and considering that "physicians often regard their perspective as better than the perspective of their religiously recalcitrant patient," coercion is tempting, but it would be both immoral and unethical and should be avoided at all cost.[550]

---

[547] See *supra* note 281 of chapter 3 and accompanying text.

[548] Spence, "The Status of Bloodless Surgery," *supra* note 508 of chapter 9.

[549] Parizeau & Carbonneau, Consentement éclairé et transfusion sanguine, *supra* note 540, 168.

[550] Thomas, "Ethical Reflections on Patient Refusals of Life-Saving Treatment," *supra* note 541, 260.

CONCLUSION

The Doctor Needs to be Informed

Patients who object to a recommended medical treatment on religious or moral grounds pose an ethical and legal challenge to health-care professionals. The challenge however, need not lead to confrontation. Consistent with the physician's responsibility to provide net medical benefit to patients with minimal harm, serious consideration must be given to the value and belief system of the patient. The physician who takes on the role of an 'informed doctor' will serve his patients well, in keeping with fundamental legal and ethical principles.

In the case of the Jehovah's Witness patient, the physician needs to understand the nature and depth of the belief. As was set out in earlier chapters, their objection is a religious one, based on their understanding of the Bible and reflecting the views of some early church writers, as well as 17th and 18th century Bible commentators. The Witnesses have published numerous articles setting out the Scriptural basis for their belief. These are available to anyone who wishes to be informed. As a further measure, they have set up liaison committees throughout the world to assist their members, and provide information to physicians concerning available alternatives.

Witnesses have also drawn attention to the near religious or 'magical' aurora which has surrounded the use of blood in the medical field since the earliest of times. Pharaohs bathed in it, epileptics drank it, whereas Galen, Patin and Rush were all convinced that without a 'good bleed' there was no chance of recovery. Bloodletting having by this time fallen into disrepute, during and after the wars of the past century the 'queen of remedies' gradually switched to blood transfusion therapy.

Physicians who practiced bloodletting, such as Benjamin Rush, were convinced that they were saving their patients when in fact, in many cases, they were hastening their death. Finally judged by the medical profession to be futile, bloodletting gave way to the practice of transfusing blood. Again, physicians hasten the death of a great many patients, this time by unknowingly (and in some case, knowingly) transfusing contaminated blood. Thus, while some physicians may continue to view blood as the 'queen of remedies', many now realize the dangerous nature of blood therapy, including its potentially lethal character. In view of the risks associated with blood transfusions, and the availability of numerous alternatives, Witnesses argue their refusal of blood therapy as reasonable from a medical viewpoint.

Initially, patients were at the mercy of the benevolent and paternalist doctor. With the emergence of bioethics, there occurred a transformation in the balance of power with patients and doctors forging a new style of relationship. Some characteristics of this new relationship, such as the rule of informed consent, were imposed by law. Still other aspects were the result of the erosion of paternalism in favor of the right of the patient to self-determination. Thus, the patient today may choose a particular medical treatment or no treatment at all. The choice belongs to the patient, and to the patient alone.

This is particularly important in the case of the patient who refuses a particular medical treatment for religious or moral reasons since the physician must address this issue from a moral viewpoint, and not a medical one. To be successful, he will need to become an 'informed doctor' as the information needed is outside the realm of medicine.

While many may continue to find it difficult to deal with the question of 'ethics, blood and God' the 'informed doctor' will be better equipped to address this issue and to respect the patient as an autonomous individual in control of his own destiny.

See footnote 263.

PAS DE TRANSFUSION SANGUINE!

En tant que témoin de Jéhovah attaché à mes convictions religieuses, je demande que l'on ne m'administre ni sang ni dérivés du sang en aucune circonstance. Je suis pleinement conscient de la portée de ma décision, mais je suis absolument résolu à obéir au commandement de la Bible qui dit de "s'abstenir (...) du sang". (Actes 15:28, 29.) Toutefois, mes croyances me permettent d'accepter des substituts non sanguins comme le Dextran, l'Haemaccel, le Plasmagel, le Plasmion et le Rhéomacrodex ou une solution saline.

Signature ____________________

Adresse ____________________

[Translation]

NO BLOOD TRANSFUSION!

As one of Jehovah's Witnesses with firm religious convictions, I request that no blood or blood products be administered to me under any circumstances. I fully realize the implications of this position, but I have resolutely decided to obey the Bible command: "Keep abstaining . . . from blood." (Acts 15:28, 29) However, I have no religious objection to use the nonblood alternatives, such as Dextran, Haemaccel, PVP, Ringer's Lactate or saline solution.

See footnote 82

NO BLOOD

MEDICAL DIRECTIVE

(signed document inside)

Medical problems: ____________________

Current medication: ____________________

Allergies: ____________________

IN CASE OF EMERGENCY, PLEASE CONTACT:

Name: ____________________

Telephone: ____________________

Address: ____________________

____

ALTERNATE CONTACT:

Name: ____________________

Telephone:

Address: ____________________

____

Open to signed document ⬇

ADVANCE MEDICAL DIRECTIVE/RELEASE

I, ____________________, make this advance directive as a formal statement of my wishes. These instructions reflect my resolute and informed decision.

I direct that ***no blood transfusions*** (whole blood, red cells, white cells, platelets, or blood plasma) be given to me under any circumstances, even if physicians deem such necessary to preserve my life or health. I will accept nonblood expanders, nonblood pharmaceuticals that control hemorrhage and stimulate the production of red blood cells, and other nonblood management.

This legal directive is an exercise of my right to accept or to refuse medical treatment in accord with my deeply held values and convictions. I am one of Jehovah's Witnesses, and I make this directive out of obedience to commands in the Bible, such as: "Keep abstaining . . . from blood." (Acts 15:28, 29) This is, and has been, my unwavering religious stand for _____ years. I am _____ years old.

I also know that there are various dangers associated with blood transfusions. So I have decided to avoid such dangers and, instead, to accept whatever risks may seem to be involved in my choice of alternative nonblood management.

I release physicians, anesthesiologists, and hospitals and their personnel from liability for any damages that might be caused by my refusal of blood, despite their otherwise competent care.

Signature ____________________

Address ____________________ Date ____________________

____________________ Telephone ____________________

Witness ____________________

Witness ____________________

md-E 6/01 Printed in Canada

BIBLIOGRAPHY

LEGISLATION

Infants Act, R.S.B.C. 1979, c. 196

Medical Consent of Minors Act, N.B. Acts, 1979, c. 41

Proposals for an Advance Health-care Directive Act, Law Reform Commission of Saskatchewan, Report to the Minister of Justice, Dec. 1991

Quebec Chart of Human Rights, 1975 (L.R.Q. c. C-12)

Quebec Civil Code, Art. 13, 14

JURISPRUDENCE

Adler v. Ontario, [1996] 3 S.C.R. 607

B. (R.) v. Children's Aid, [1995] 1 S.C.R. 315

Bennan v. Parsonnet (1912), 83 N.J.L.R. 20

Boyer v. Grignon, [1988] R.J.Q. 829

Caron v. Gagnon, (1930) R.J. 155 (S. Ct.)

Chaput v. Romain, [1955] S.C.R. 834

Crouse Irving Memorila Hospital, Inc. v. Paddock, 127 Misc. 2d 101, 485 N.Y.S.2d 433 (Sup. Ct. Onondaga County 1985)

Dobson (Litigation Guardian of) v. Dobson, Supreme Court of Canada, File No. 26152, December 8, 1999: July 9

Evelyn Estrella v. Princess Margaret Hospital, June 2, 1999, Court. File No. 99-CV-170514

Fosmire v. Nicoleau, 551 N.E.2d 77

Fosmire v. Nicoleau, 75 N.Y.2d 218, 551 N.E.2d 77, 551 N.Y.S.2d 876 (1990), 144 A.D.2d 8, 536 N.Y.S.2d 492 (1989)

Holmes v. Silver Cross Hosp. 340 F. Supp. 125 (N.D. Ill 1972)

Hopp v. Lepp, [1980] 2 S.C.R. 192

In re Brooks, 32 Ill. 2d 361, 205 N.E.2d 435 (1965)

In re Dubreuil, 629 So. 2d 819 (Fla. 1993), 603 So. 2d 538 (Fla. Dist. Ct. App. 1992)

In re Estate of Dorone, 502 A.2d 1271 (Pa. Super. 1985)

In re Harrell, 678 So. 2d 455 (Fla. Dist. Ct. App. 1996)

In re Huges, 259 N.J. Super. 193, 611 a.2d 1148 (App. Div. 1992)

In re Jamaica Hospital, 128 Misc. 2d 1006, 491 N.Y.S.2d 898 (Sup. Ct. Queens County 1985)

In re Melideo, 88 Misc. 2d 974, 390 N.Y.S.2d 523 (Sup. Ct. 1976)

In re Osborne, 294 A.2d 372, 376 n.6 (D.C. 1972)

In re President and Directors of Georgetown College 331 F.2d 1000 (Wright, J., in chambers), 331 F.2d 1010 (D.C. Cir.) cert. Denied, 377 U.S. 978 (1964)

In re President and Directors of Georgetown College, 331 F.2d 1010

In re Quackenbush, 156 N.J. Super. 282, 383 A2d 785 (1978)

In re Quinlan, 70 N.J. 10, 355 A.2d 647 (1976) 617

In re Rena, 705 N.E.2d 1155 (Mass. Ct. App. 1999)

In re W.M., 823 S.W. 2d 128 (Mo. Ct. App. 1992)

In re Winthrop University Hospital, 128 Misc. 2d 804, 490 N.Y.S.2d 996 (Sup. Ct. Nassau County 1985)

Kenney v. Lockwood Clinic Ltd., (1931) 4 D.L.R. 906, O.R. 438; rev. (1932), 1 D.L.R. 507 O.R. 141 (Ontario)

Lakeshore General Hospital v. Methot-Gaudreault, Sup. Ct. Montreal, no. 500-05-008750-844, August 1, 1984

Malette v. Shulman et al., 63 O.R. (2d) 243 (Ont. Sup. Ct., 1987)

Malette v. Shulman, 67 D.L.R. (4th) 321 (Ont. C.A. 1990)

Manoir de la Pointe Bleue (1978) Inc. v. Corbeil, [1992] R.J.Q. 712 (S. Ct.)

Marshall v. Curry (1933), 3 D.L.R. 60 Can. C.C. 136 (Nova Scotia)

Marshall v. Curry (1933), 3 D.L.R. 260 (N.S.S.C)

McKenzie v. Doctors' Hosp. of Hollywood, Inc., 765 F. Supp. 1504, 1505 (S.D. Fla. 1991)

Mercy Hosp., Inc. v. Jackson, 489 A.2d 1130 (Md. Ct. Spec. App. 1985)

Mulloy v. Hop Sang, (1935) 1 W.W.R. 714

Murray v. McMurchy (1949), 2 D.L.R. 442

Norwood Hospital v. Munoz, 409 Mass. 116, 564 H.E.2d 1017 (1991)

Norwood Hospital v. Munoz, 564 N.E. 2d 1017 (Mass. 1991)

Olmstead v. US, 277 US 472 (1927)

Parmley v. Parmley, [1945] 4 D.L.R. 81 (S.C.C.)

Pittman v. Bain, [1994] 19 C.C.L.T. (2d) 1 (Ont. Ct. Gen. Div.)

Powell v. Columbian Presbyterian medical Center, 49 Miscf. 2d 215, 267 N.Y.S.2d 450 (Sup. Ct. N.Y. County 1965)

Public Health Trust v. Wons, 541 So. 2d 96 (Fla. 1989), 500 So. 2d at 679 (Fla. Dist. Ct. App. 1987)

Re A.Y., 111 348 A.P.R. 91 (Nfld. Fam. Ct. 1993)

Re L.D.K., 48 R.F.L. (2d) 164 (Ont. Prov. Ct.)

Re L.D.K.; C.A.S. v. K. (1985) 48 R.F.L. (2d) 164 (Ont. Prov. Ct.)

Region 2 Hospital Corp. v. Walker, 4 R.F.L. (4th) 321 (New Brunswick Ct. App. 1994)

Reibl v. Hughes, [1980] 2 S.C.R. 180

Schloendorff v. Society of New York Hospital, (1914), 211 N. Y. 125

Slater v. Baker (1767) 2 Wils. K.B. 359, 95 E.R. 860; 22 Hals. (2nd ed.) 319

Superintendent of Belchertown State School v. Saikewicz, Mass. 370 N.E. 2d 417 (1977)

U.S. v. Garber, 589 F. 2d 843 (5th Cir. 1979)

United States v. George, 239 F. Supp. 752 (D. Conn. 1965)

Weiss c. Solomon, [1989] R.J.Q. 731 (S. Ct.)

Werth v. Taylor, 475 N.W.2d 426 (Mich. Ct. App. 1991)

Winn v. Alexander and the Soldiers' Memorial Hospital, (1940) O.W.N. 238

BOOKS

1999 Yearbook of Jehovah's Witnesses. New York: Watch Tower Bible and Tract Society of New York 1999

A.M.S. Le refus des transfusions sanguines. Guyancourt: A.M.S. 1990

Annas, G. & al. The Nazi Doctors and the Nuremberg Code. New York: Oxford University Press 1992

Arnold, E. The Early Christians After the Death of the Apostles. New York: Plough Publishing House 1972

Beauchamp, T., & al. Principles of Biomedical Ethics. New York: Oxford University Press 1994

Bendixen, H. H. "Preface" in Blood and Blood Products. Washington: National Academy Press 1996

Benson, J. The Holy Bible, Containing the Old and New Testaments. New York: 1839

Binns, L. E. Innocent III. London: Methuen & Co. Ltd. 1931

Boyd, K. "Moral and Religious Dilemmas" in Critical Care – Standards, Audit and Ethics. London: Arnold 1996

Brock, D. "Death and Dying" in Medical Ethics. Boston: Jones and Bartlett 1997

Brockliss, L. & Jones, C. The Medical World of Early Modern France. Oxford: Clarendon Press 1997

Burton-Bradley, B. G. A History of Medicine in Papua New Guinea. Kingsgrove: Australasian Medical publishing Company Limited 1990

Butterfield, L. H., ed., Letters of Benjamin Rush, 1793-1813, vol. II. Princeton, N.J.: Princeton University Press 1951

Calhoune, L. "Blood Product Preparation and Administration" in Clinical Practice of Transfusion Medicine, 3d. ed. New York: Churchill Livingstone 1995

Callahan, D. The Sanctity of Life. Boston: Beacon Press 1968

Calvin, J. Commentaries on the First Book of Moses Called Genesis. Edinburgh: The Edinburgh Printing Company 1847

Capland, A., ed. When Medicine Went Mad: Bioethics and the Holocaust. Totowa: Humana Press 1992

Catholic Hospital Association. Religious Aspects of Medical Care: A Handbook of Religious Practices of All Faiths. St-Louis: The Catholic Hospital Association 1978

Childress, J. "The Normative Principles of Medical Ethics" in Medical Ethics. Boston: Jones and Bartlett 1997

Clarke, A. The Holy Bible, Containing the Old and New Testaments. New York: Carlton & Porter 1856

Clarke, A. The New Testament of our Lord and Savior Jesus Christ. New York: Carlton & Phillips 1856

Crosby, H. The New Testament in Both Authorized and Revised Versions. Boston: Carles F. Alden & Company 1884

Dalderby, J. The Ecclesiastical History of the Second and Third Centuries. London: Francis & John Rivington 1845

Davis, J. D. The Westminster Dictionary of the Bible. Philadelphia: The Westminster Press 1944

Delitzsch, F. A New Commentary on Genesis. Edinburgh: T. & T. Clark 1888

Dierkens, R. Les droits sur le corps et le cadavre de l'homme. Paris: Masson et Cie 1996

Dods, M. The Works of Aurelius Augustine, Bishop of Hippo, vol. V. Edinburgh: T. & T. Clark 1822

Driver, S. R. The Book of Genesis. London: Methuen & Co. 1904

Ellis, P. J. Transfusion Therapy, Principles and Procedures. Rockville: Aspen Systems Corporation 1981

Emson, H. The Doctor and the Law. Toronto: Butterworths Canada 1989

Engelhardt, H. The Foundations of Bioethics. Oxford: Oxford University Press 1996

Eusebius. An Ecclesiastical History, trans. Cruse, C.F. Samuel Bagster and Sons, Paternoster Row 1842

Fakhry, I., & al. "Blood Transfusions and Disorders or Surgical Bleeding" in Textbook of Surgery. Philadelphia: W.B. Saunders 1997

Family Care and Medical Management for Jehovah's Witnesses. New York: Watchtower Bible and Tract Society of New York 1995

Farr, A.D. God, Blood and Society. Aberdeen: Impulse Publications Ltd. 1972

Fleming, A. Medical Milestones. Baltimore: The Williams & Wilkins Co. 1952

Flint, A. Practice of Medicine. Philadelphia: Henry C. Lea's Son and Company 1881

Fuller, A. G. Complete Works of the Rev. Andrew Fuller, with a Memoir of his life. London: G. & J. Dyer, Paternoster Row 1846

Garrison, F. H. An Introduction to the History of Medicine. London: W. B. Saunders Company 1929

Gilmartin, G. "Jehovah's Witnesses" in Ethical Issues in Anaesthesia. Oxford: Butterworth-Heinemann 1994

Graffard, S., & al. Les Bibelforscher et le nazisme (1933-1945) Ces oubliés de l'Histoire. Paris: Editions TIRESIAS 1991

Grisso, T. Evaluating Competencies – Forensic Assessments and Instruments. New York: Plenum Press 1986

Gruber, U. F. Blood Replacement. Heidelberg: Springer-Verlag Berlin 1969

Guiou, N. M. Transfusion, A Canadian Surgeon's Story in War and in Peace. Yarmouth: Stoneycroft Publishing 1985

Hall, S. G. Women Among the Early Martyrs in Martyrs and Martyrologies. Oxford: Blackwell Publishers 1993

Halsted, W. S. Surgical Papers. Baltimore: Johns Hopkins Press 1924

Hastings, J., ed. Dictionary of the Bible. New York: Charles Scribner's Sons 1963

Héritier, J. La sève de l'homme. Paris: Éditions Denoël 1987

Houdre, J.-P. Aperçu sur l'historique de la transfusion sanguine depuis les origines jusqu'au XIXème siècle. Paris: L'imprimerie R. Foulon & Cie 1968

How Can Blood Save Your Life? Georgetown: Watch Tower Bible and Tract Society of Canada 1990

Illich, I. Limits to Medicine. Toronto: McClelland & Steward Ltd. 1976

Institute of Medicine, HIV and the Blood Supply: An Analysis of Critical Decisionmaking. Washington: National Academy Press 1995

Is there a Creator Who Cares About You? New York: Watchtower Bible and Tract Society of New York, Inc. 1998

Ispahany, B. Islamic Medical Wisdom The Tibb Al-A'Imma. London: The Muhammadi Trust of Great Britain and Northern Ireland 1991

Jehovah's Witnesses in the Twentieth Century. Georgetown: Watch Tower Bible and Tract Society of Canada 1989

Joseph, N., & al. "Blood Salvage Techniques" in Blood Conservation in the Surgical Patient. Baltimore: Williams & Wilkins 1996

Kant, E. "Groundwork of the Metaphysics of Morals" in Immanuel Kant, Practical Philosophy. Cambridge: Cambridge University Press 1996

Kaplan, W. State and Salvation - The Jehovah's Witnesses and Their Fight for Civil Rights. Toronto: University of Toronto Press 1989

Kevy & Gorlin "Red Cell Transfusion" in Hematology of Infancy and Childhood, 5th ed. Philadelphia: W.B. Saunders 1998

Keyserlingk, E. Sanctity of Life or Quality of Life. Ottawa: Minister of Supply and Services Canada 1979

Khushf, G. "The Sanctity of Life: A Literature Review" in Sanctity of Life and Human Dignity. Dordrecht: Kluwer Academic 1996

King, L. S. Medical Thinking – A Historical Preface. Princeton: Princeton University Press 1982

Knowledge That Leads to Everlasting Life. New York: Watch Tower Bible and Tract Society of New York, Inc. 1995

Krever, H. "Interim Report" in Commission of Inquiry of the Blood System in Canada. Ottawa: Canada Communication Group 1995

Kuhse, H. The Sanctity-of-Life Doctrine in Medicine. Oxford: Clarendon Press 1987

L'Ancien, P., trans. Ernout, A. Histoire naturelle. Paris: Société d'édition "Les belles lettres" 1962

Lang, D., & al. "Blood Conservation in Jehovah's Witnesses" in Blood Conservation in the Surgical Patient. Baltimore: Williams & Wilkins 1996

Lifton, R. The Nazi Doctor: Medical Killing and the Psychology of Genocide. New York: Basic Books 1986

Luther's Works (Church and Ministry III) (E. Gritsch ed. N.d.)

Masson, A. H.B. History of the Blood Transfusion Service in Edinburgh. Edinburgh: Alastair H. B. Masson 1993

Mayrand, A. L'inviolabité de la personne humaine. Montreal: Wilson & Lafleur 1975

McCullough, J. Transfusion Medicine. New York: McGraw-Hill 1998

McDuff, J. Le sang qui tue. Montreal: Libre expression 1995

McGarvey, J. W. A Commentary on Acts of Apostles. Lexington: Transylvania Printing and Publishing Co. 1872

Mill, J. S. "On Liberty" in Essential Works of John Stuart Mill. New York: Bantam Books 1965

Miller, W.V. "Adverse Effects of Blood Transfusion" in Transfusion Therapy, Principles and Procedures. Rockville: Aspen Systems Corporation 1981

Milner, J. The History of the Church of Christ. London: Thomas Cadell, In the Strand 1834

Moeller, W. History of the Christian Church AD 1-600. New York: The Macmillan Co. 1902

Mollinson, P. L., Engelfriet, C. P. & Contreras, M. Blood Transfusion in Clinical Medicine, 9th ed. Oxford: Blackwell Scientific Publications 1993

New International Version of The Holy Bible. East Brunswick, New Jersey: International Bible Society 1984

Newton, I. The Chronology of Ancient Kingdoms Amended. London: Printed for J. Tonson, J. Osborn and T. Longman 1728

Oberman, H.A. "The History of Transfusion Medicine" in Clinical Practice of Transfusion Medicine, 3rd ed. New York: Churchill Livingstone 1995

Organized to Accomplish Our Ministry. New York: Watch Tower Bible and Tract Society of New York 1989

Oritz de Montellano, B. R. Aztec Medicine, Health and Nutrition. London: Rutgers University Press 1990

Osler, W. & McCrae, T. The Principles and Practice of Medicine. New York: D. Appleton and Company 1920

Parizeau M.-H. et Carbonneau, A. "Analyse éthique du consentement à l'acte transfusionnel et repères juridiques dans le contexte canadien et québécois," in Consentement éclairé et transfusion sanguine. Rennes: Éditions ENSP 1996

Pellegrino, E. "Toward an Expanded Medical Ethics: The Hippocratic Ethic Revisited" in Hippocrates Revisited a Search for Meaning. New York: Medcom Press 1973

Penmery, J.-J. Les Origines de la transfusion sanguine. Amsterdam: B. M. Israel N. V. 1974

Percival, H.R. The Seven Ecumenical Councils of the Undivided Church, vol. XIV. New York: Charles Scribner's Sons 1900

Picard, A. The Gift of Death. Toronto: HarperCollins Publisher Ltd. 1995

Pichon, J. Le Ménagier de Paris, vol. I. Paris: Société des bibliophiles français 1846

Pirie, A. A Dissertation on Baptism and Letters on the Sinai Covenant; Together with an Inquiry into the Lawfulness of Eating Blood. Edinburgh: J. Pillans & Sons, Lawnmarket 1806

Porter, R. The Greatest Benefit to Mankind. New York: W. W. Norton & Company 1997

Ramsey, P. "The Morality of Abortion" in Moral Problems: A Collection of Philosophical Essays. New York: Harper & Row 1971

Ramsey, P. The Patient as a Person. London: Yale University Press 1972

Roberts, A. & Donaldson, J. The Ante-Nicene Fathers. Translations of The Writings of the Fathers down to AD 325. New York: Charles Scribner's Sons 1925

Robinson, C. H. The Life of Otto Apostle of Pomerania. New York: The Macmillan Company 1920

Rossi, E. C., Simon, T. L. & Moss, G. S. Principles of Transfusion Medicine. Baltimore: Williams & Wilkins 1991

Rothman, D. Strangers at the Bedside. New York: Basic Books 1991

Rozovsky, L., & al. The Canadian Law of Consent to Treatment. Toronto: Butterworths Canada 1990

Rozovsky, L. Canadian Hospital Law. Toronto: Canadian Hospital Association 1974

Rutkow, I. M. American Surgery, An Illustrated History. New York: Lippincott-Raven 1998

Sazama, K. "Adverse Effects of Blood Transfusions" in Conn's Current Therapy. Philidelphia: Saunders 1999

Schaff, P. & Wace, H. A select Library of Nicene and Post-Nicene Fathers, vol. II. New York: The Christian Literature Company 1894

Sharma, P. V. History of Medicine in India from Antiquity to 1000 AD New Delhi: Indian National Science Academy 1992

Shils, E. "The Sanctity of Life" in Life or Death: Ethics and Options. Seattle: University of Washington Press 1968

Smith, W. A Dictionary of the Bible. Chicago: The John C. Winston Company 1884

Soloman. "A History of Transfusion Medicine" in III American Association Blood Banks, Administrative Manual. A. Ross ed. 1990

Sommerville, A. Medical Ethics Today: Its Practice and Philosophy. London: B.M.J. Publishing Group 1993

Spence, R. K. "Management of Surgical Patients with Special Problems" in Clinical Practice of Transfusion Medicine, 3d ed. New York: Churchill Livingstone 1995

Spence, R.K. "Beneficial Aspects of Surgical Transfusion" in Blood and Blood Products: Safety and Risk. Washington: National Academy Press 1996

Spence, R. K. "Blood Saving Strategies in Surgical Patients," in Clinical Practice of Transfusion Medicine, 3rd edition. New York: Churchill Livingstone 1995

Spencer, W.G. (trans.). Celsus de Medicina. Cambridge: Harvard University Press 1960

Starr, D. Blood, An Epic History of Medicine and Commerce. New York: Alfrede A. Knopf 1998

Stevens, C.E. "The Epidemiology of Non-A Non-B Hepatitis in the United States" in Blood Transfusion, Blood Components and Hepatitis, Second USA-USSR Joint Symposium, Bethesda, Maryland, 24-26 September 1979. U.S. Department of Health and Human Services 1980

Swisher & Petz. Overview and General Principles of Transfusion Medicine: Clinical Practice of Transfusion Medicine, 3d ed. New York: Churchill Livingstone 1996

Tannahill, R. Flesh & Blood. London: Abacus 1996

Tertullian Apologetical Works and Minucius Felix Octavius, transl. R. Arbesmann, et al. Washington: The Catholic University of America Press, Inc. 1950

The Bible, God's Word or Man's? New York: Watchtower Bible and Tract Society of New York, Inc. 1989

The Royal College of Surgeons of England, Code of Practice for the Surgical Management of Jehovah's Witnesses. London: The Royal College of Surgeons of England 1996

Titmuss, R. M. The Gift Relationship. London: George Alloen & Unwin Ltd. 1970

True Peace and Security – How Can You Find It? New York: Watchtower Bible and Tract Society of New York, Inc. 1977

Veatch, R. "Medical Ethics, An Introduction" in Medical Ethics. Boston: Jones and Bartlett 1997

Verhey, A. "Scripture and Medical Ethics: Psalm 51:10A, The Jarvik VII, and Psalm 50:9" in Religious Methods and Resources in Bioethics, ed. by P. Camenisch. Boston: Kluwer Academic 1994

Wailoo, K. Drawing Blood. Baltimore: The Johns Hopkins University Press 1997

Wesley, J. Explanatory Notes upon the New Testament. London: Wesleyan Conference Office 1754

Williams, G. The Sanctity of Life and Criminal Law. London: Faber and Faber 1958

Wilson, B. "Complications of Blood Transfusions" in Complications in Surgery and Their Management. Philadelphia: Saunders 1961

Wolf & Gold. "Current Practice of Blood Transfusion in Cardiac Surgery" in Blood Conservation in Cardiac Surgery. New York: Springer 1998

You Can Live Forever in Paradise on Earth. New York: Watch Tower Bible and Tract Society of New York 1989

JOURNALS AND CONFERENCES

Watchtower Society journals:

"An 'Exclusion Clause' Recommended" The Watchtower (15 December 1950): 524

"Early Christians Under Roman Rule" The Watchtower (1 March 1951): 137

"Are Blood Transfusions Really Necessary?" Awake! (22 August 1999): 31

"Baptism" The Watchtower (1 August 1958): 472

"Be Faithful to God 'Who Looks On in Secret'" The Watchtower (15 April 1985): 12

"Blood Transfusion – One Doctor's Opinion" Awake! (8 January 1949): 12

"Blood Transfusions: Why Many are Taking a Fresh Look" Awake! (8 September 1978): 16

"'Bread of Life' Available for All" The Watchtower (15 February 1986): 18

"Bridging the Gap Between Doctors and Witness Patients" Awake! (22 November 1990): 21

"Bullfighting – Art or Outrage?" Awake! (8 July 1990): 19

"By Man's Way or by God's Way – Which?" The Watchtower (1 December 1967): 721

"Canada's 'Tainted Blood' Inquiry" Awake! (8 June 1995): 20

"Dangers of Blood Transfusion" Awake! (22 October 1948): 12

"Doctor-Patient Communication – A Key To Success" Awake! (8 March 1991): 12

"Doctors Take a New Look at Bloodless Surgery" Awake! (8 December 1998): 18

"Doing What We Can to Maintain a Better Life" Awake! (22 April 1977): 6

"Elders, Judge with Righteousness" The Watchtower (1 July 1992): 19

"Euthanasia and God's Law" The Watchtower (15 February 1961): 118

"Facing Up to Questions of Conscience" The Watchtower (1 October 1972): 589

"Gaining Peace with God Through Dedication and Baptism" The Watchtower (15 April 1987): 12

"How Precious Is Life to You?" The Watchtower (15 January 1995): 3

"Immovable for the Right Worship" The Watchtower (1 July 1945): 195

"Is Blood Transfusion Scriptural?" Awake! (22 September 1949): 25

"Jehovah's Witnesses and the Medical Profession Cooperate" Awake! (22 November 1993): 24

"Keep on Walking in Jehovah's Way" The Watchtower (15 May 1999): 19

"Keeping God's Congregation Clean in the Time of His Judgment" The Watchtower (1 June 1973): 339

"Le Sang" La Recherche 24 (May 1993)

"Medical Alternatives to Blood Transfusions" (Report of proceedings and recommendations of conference *Building a Blood System in the 21st Century*, Toronto, 3-4 November 1997) (1997) Hospital Information Services (Canada) for Jehovah's Witnesses: 57

"Mercy Killing – What Do Lawyers Say?" Awake! (8 March 1978): 7

"Motorcycles – How Dangerous Are They?" Awake! (8 April 1992): 10

"My Life With Hemophilia" Awake! (22 June 1987): 21

"My Ten Years in Spain's Military Prisons" The Watchtower (1 October 1985): 19

"Nonblood Treatment – What Experts Say" Awake! (8 March 1999): 19

"One Reason for God's Vengeance" The Watchtower (15 December 1927): 376

"Pioneering Bloodless Surgery with Jehovah's Witnesses" Awake! (8 March 1991): 12

"Respect for the Sanctity of Blood" The Watchtower (15 September 1961): 553

"Seminars to Improve Relations Between Doctors and Jehovah's Witnesses" Awake! (22 March 1995): 19

"Settling Doctrinal Differences" Zion's Watch Tower (15 April 1909): 117

"Should Babies Be Baptized?" The Watchtower (15 March 1986): 7

"Should You Be Baptized?" The Watchtower (1 April 1993): 4

"The Apostolic Council" Zion's Watch Tower (15 November 1892): 350

"The Christian Congregation and Its Operation" The Watchtower (1 October 1977): 600

"The Most Precious Fluid in the World" Awake! (22 October 1990): 15

"Thrill Sports – Should I Take a Chance?" Awake! (8 July 1994): 9

"Treasure the Real Life" The Watchtower (15 January 1995): 6

"Walk as Instructed by Jehovah" The Watchtower (15 June 1991): 13

"Water Safety Is No Accident" Awake! (22 May 1988): 15

"Why the Rise in Suicide?" Awake! (8 August 1975): 25

"Question From Readers - Are we to consider the injection of serums such as diphtheria toxin antitoxin and blood fractions such as gamma globulin into the blood stream, for the purpose of building up resistance to disease by means of antibodies, the same as the drinking of blood or the taking of blood or blood plasma by means of transfusion?—N. P., United States." The Watchtower (15 September 1958): 575

"Question From Readers - Although it is unscriptural for a Christian to accept another person's blood in transfusion, would it be allowable for a dedicated Christian to have some of his own blood removed and then put back into his body during an operation?—W. D., U.S.A." The Watchtower (15 October 1959): 640

"Question From Readers - In view of the seriousness of taking blood into the human system by a transfusion, would violation of the Holy Scriptures in this regard subject the dedicated, baptized receiver of blood transfusion to being disfellowshiped from the Christian congregation?" The Watchtower (15 January 1961): 63

"Question From Readers - How can one tell if meat purchased from a butcher or in some other market has been properly bled? Also, how can one tell if cold-meat loaves, pastry or preparations sold by druggists contain any blood or blood fractions?—A. R., U.S.A.; How can we harmonize the Scriptural counsel, "Everything that is sold in a meat market keep eating, making no inquiry on account of your conscience" (1 Cor. 10:25), with the advice recently contained in *The Watchtower,* to make reasonable inquiry at places where one buys meat to be sure that it has been properly bled? (*The Watchtower,* September 15, 1961, page 557)—N. Q., U.S.A.; In view of the Bible command on abstinence from blood, how are fish and insects to be prepared in order to be acceptable for food?—B. F., U.S.A; Since the Bible forbids the eating of blood, how are Christians to view the use of serums and vaccines? Has the Society changed its viewpoint on this?—J. D., U.S.A." The Watchtower (1 November 1961): 669

"Question From Readers – Does a substantial health danger justify having an abortion?" The Watchtower (15 March 1975): 191

"Question From Readers - Do Jehovah's Witnesses allow the use of autologous blood (autotransfusion), such as by having their own blood stored and later put back into them?" The Watchtower (1 March 1989): 30

"Question From Readers – Do Jehovah's Witnesses accept injections of a blood fraction, such as immune globulin or albumin?" The Watchtower (1 June 1990): 31

"Question From Readers - How strenuously should a Christian resist a blood transfusion that has been ordered or authorized by a court?" The Watchtower

(15 June 1991): 31

"Question From Readers - Would it be proper to accept a vaccination or some other medical injection containing albumin derived from human blood?" The Watchtower (1 October 1994): 31

"Question From Readers - Do Jehovah's Witnesses accept any medical products derived from blood?" The Watchtower (15 June 2000): 30

"Question Form Readers – In the light of Bible commands about the proper use of blood, how do Jehovah's Witnesses view medical procedures using one's own blood?" The Watchtower (15 October 2000): 30

Other journals:

ABC NEWS, 20/20 aired on 19 March 1987, hosts Hugh Downs & Barbara Walters, producer Joseph R. Lovett and correspondent Tom Jarriel.

Adams, J. "Respecting the Right to Be Wrong" (1998) 5 Acad. Emerg. Med.. 753

Alexander, L. "Medical Science Under Dictatorship" (1949) 241 New Eng. J. of Med.: 39

Andrews, L. "Legal, Ethical, and Medical Guidelines for Jehovah's Witnessses in Surgery" (1979) 34 Week. Anest. Upd. 1

Argy, O. "Another Standare of Care – Patient, In Reply" 276:6 JAMA: 450

Atighetchi, D. "Bioethics and Islam" in Proceedings of the 10th World Congress on Medical Law, Jerusalem (Israel) Aug. (1994): 26

Baron, C.H. "Blood, Sin, and Death: Jehovah's Witnesses and the American Patients' Rights Movement" (Colloquim on "Sang et droit", University of Paris X (Nanterre), 14-15 May 1993)

Bartholome, W. "A Revolution in Understanding: How Ethics Has Transformed Health-care Decision Making" (1992) Qual. Rev. Bull.: 9

Beeson, P.B. "Jaundice Occurring One to Four Months After Transfusion of Blood or Plasma" (1943) 121 JAMA: 1332

Blajchman, M.A. "Transfusion-Related Issues in Jehovah's Witness Patients" (1991) V Trans. Med Rev.: 243

Bleecher, H. "Ethics and Clinical Research" (1966) 274 NEJM: 1354

Blundell, J. "Experiments on the Transfusion of Blood by the Syringe" (1818) IX

Medico-Chir. Tr.: 56

Blundell, J. "Some Accounts of a Case of Obstinate Vomiting in which an Attempt was Made to Prolong Life by the Injection of Blood Into the Veins" (1818) X Medico-Chir. Tr.: 310

Bonakdar, M. I. & al. Major Gynecologic and Obstetric surgery on Jehovah's Witnesses" (November 1982) 60:5 Obst. & Gyn.: 587

Bragg, R. "Fake Witnesses Avoid Transfusions" The Toronto Star (25 February 1997): A9

Bryan, L. Jr. "Blood-Letting in American Medicine, 1830-1892" (1964) 38 Bull. Of the Hist. Of Med.: 516

Bueckert, D. "Bloodless Medicine Continuing to Gain in Popularity" The Globe and Mail (4 January 1997): A10

Burns, J. M. "When Patients Refuse Blood Transfusion: Meeting the Medical and Legal Challenge" (1997) 3 Advances in Legal Med.: 261

Capen, K. "Informed Consent and Blood Transfusions: What does Krever's Interim Report Mean to Doctors?" (1995) 152 Can. Med. Assoc. J.:1663

Carlson, D.-L. "Clients Living Proof of Canada's Tainted-Blood Scandal" (13-19 June 1994) Law Times: 4

Chown, B. "Transfusions are Dangerous" (1 December 1957) 77 Can. M. A. J.: 1037

Clay, M. A. "Ethical and Legal Implications of Bloodless Medicine and Surgery" (1999) 14:1 J. Intensive Care Med.: 34

Clouser, K. "The Sanctity of Life: An Analysis of a Concept" (1973) 78 Ann. of Med. Eth.: 165

"Compte rendu du colloque de Bordeaux du 8 novembre 1986" (1986)

"Consensus Conference: Blood Management-Surgical Practice Guidelines" (1995) 170 Amer. J. of Surg.: 1S

Cooley, D.A. & al. "Open Heart Surgery in Jehovah's Witnesses" (June 1964) 13 Amer. J. of Card.: 779

Cooper, J., Jr. "Perioperative Considerations in Jehovah's Witnesses" (1990) 28:4 Internat. Anesthesiol. Clinics: 210

Crosby, W. H. "Misuse of Blood Transfusions" (December 1958) Blood: 1198

Curran, J. & al. "Acquired Immunodeficiency Syndrome (AIDS) Associated with Transfusions" (12 January 1984) New Eng. J. of Med.: 69

Davis, S. "The Refusal of Life-Saving Medical Treatment vs. the State's Interest in the Preservation of Life: A Clarification of the Interests at Stake" (1980) 58 Wash. Univ. Law Quarterly: 85

DeCastro, R. "Bloodless Surgery: Establishment of a Program for the Special Medical Needs of the Jehovah's Witness Community—The Gynecologic Surgery Experience at a Community Hospital" (1999) 180 Am. J. Obstet. Gynecol.: 1491

Delmas, D. & Garay, A. "Le Bureau d'information Hospitalier des Témoins de Jéhovah" (July 1993) no. 88 La Gaz. de la Tranf.: 36

Devine, R. "Save the Body, Lose the Soul" (1989) Heal. Prog.: 68

Diamond, L. K. "History of Blood Banking in the United States" (1965) 193 JAMA: 40

Dickens, B. "Medical Priority of Patient's Wishes" (1991) 7:1 Humane Medicine: 7

Dixon, J. "Blood: Whose Choice and Whose Conscience" (1988) 88 N.Y St. J. of Med.: 463

Dobroszcki, J., & al. "A Cluster of Transfusion-Associated Babesiosis Cases Traced to a Single Asymptomatic Donor" (1999) 281 JAMA: 927

Dougherty, K. "La fin des transfusions?" L'Actualité (1 May 1999): 18

Downie, J. "Where There is a Will, The May Be a Better Way: Legislating Advanced Directives" (1992) 12 Health Law in Can.: 73

Drane, J. "Competency to Give an Informed Consent: A Model for Making Clinical Assessments" (1984) 252 JAMA: 925

Duh, S. "Physician Reaction to Refusal of Blood Transfusions by Jehovah's Witnesses" (1987) 79 J. Nat. Med. Assoc.: 467

Duma, H. "Bambin opéré sans transfusion sanguine" La Presse (4 February 1999): A14

Editorial (1984) 2 Lan.: 1434

Elliot, C. "Second Opinions: a Right or a Concession?" (1995) 311 B.M.J.: 671

Ellison & Silberstein "A Commentary on Three Consensus Development Conferences on Transfusion Medicine" (1990) 8 Anest. Clin. No. Am.: 624

Ely, E.W. & Bernard, G.R. "Transfusions in Critically Ill Patients" (11 February 1999) 340:6 New Eng. J. of Med.: 468

Estes, J. W. "George Washington and the Doctors: Treating America's First Superhero" (January-February 1985) Med. Her.: 43

Ferdinand, R. "Jehovah's Witnesses and Advance Directives" (1996) 96 A.J.N.: 64

Findley, L. "Blood Transfusion in Adult Jehovah's Witnesses, A Case Study of One Congregation" (1982) 142 Arch. Intern. Med.: 606

Ford, J. "The Refusal of Blood Transfusions by Jehovah's Witnesses" (1955) Feb. Linacre Quarterly: 3

Freedman, B. "A Moral Theory of Consent" (1975) 5 Hastings Cen. Rep.: 5

Garay, A. & Goni, P. "La valeur juridique de l'attestation de refus de transfusion sanguine" (13 August 1993) no. 97: 14

Garcia, F., Juri, H., Lapin, R. "Anemia and Anesthesia" (1986) 4 J. of Blood. Med. and Surg.: 15

Garrison, F.H. "The History of Bloodletting" (1 March 1913) N.Y. Med. J. 432

Gattellari, M., & al. "Informed Consent: What Did the Doctor Say?" (1999) 353 The Lancet: 1713

Gillett, G. "Learning to Do No Harm" (1993) 18 J. of Med. and Philos.: 264

Gillon, R. "Medical Ethics: Four Principles Plus Attention to Scope" (1994) 306 Brit. Med. J.: 185

Gilmore, A. "Sanctity of Life Versus Quality of Life – The Continuing Debate" (1984) 130 Can. Med. Assoc. J.: 181

Grainger, B. "Legal and Ethical Considerations in Blood Transfusion" (1997) 156:11 Can. Med. Assoc. J.: 550

Green, M. "Biblical Laws Relating to Blood Transfusion: The Judaic Laws and Principles" (1991) V Trans. Med. Rev.: 247

Grzelak, I., & al. "Blood Transfusions Downregulate Hematopoiesis and Subsequently Downregulate the Immune Response" (1998) 38 Trans.: 1104

Haug, M., & al. "Practitioner or Patient – Who's in Charge?" (1981) 22 J. of Heal. and Soc. Behav.: 215

Hebert, P. C. & al. "A Multicenter Randomized, Controlled Clinical Trial of Transfusion Requirements in Critical Care" (11 February 1999) 40:6 New Eng. J. of

Med.: 409

Henry, M. "Emergency treatment of Jehovah's Witnesses" (1991) 80 South African Med. J.: 626

Higginson, A. "Report of Seven Cases of Transfusion of Blood, With a Description of the Instrument Invented by the Author" Liverpool Medical and Chirurgical Journal 1 (1857): 102

Horty, J., Esq. "Informed Consent: Patient Can Set Limits" (1992) 8 OR Manager: 16

How, W. G. "Religion, Medicine and Law" (October 1960) Can. Bar J.: 365

Howe, E. "Influencing a Patient's Religious Beliefs: Mandate or No-Man's Land?" (1995) 6 J. Clinical Ethics: 194

Ingelfinger, F. "Informed (But Uneducated) Consent" (1972) 287 New Eng. J. of Med.: 465

Ivy, A. "Nazi War Crimes of a Medical Nature" (1949) 139 JAMA: 131

"Jehovah's Witnesses and the Question of Blood" TheWatchtower Bible and Tract Society of New York, Inc. (1977): 10

Jenish, D. "Bad Blood" Maclean's (19 September 1994): 22

Jonas, H., "Philosophical Reflections on Experimenting with Human Subjects" (1969) 98 Daedalus: 219

Jones, H. W. & Mackmull, G. "The Influence of James Blundell on the Development of Blood Transfusion" (1928) Ann. of Med. Hist.: 244

Jonsen "Blood Transfusions and Jehovah's Witnesses" (1986) 2 Clin. Car. Clin.: 97

Kambouris, A. A. "Major Abdominal Operations on Jehovah's Witnesses" (June 1987) 53 The Am. Surg.: 350

Katz, M. "Psychiatric Consultation for Competency to Refuse Medical Treatment" (1995) 36 Psychosomatics: 34

Kay, J. H. "Need for Blood in Open Heart Surgery" (3 December 1973) 226:10 JAMA: 1230

Kitchens, C. "Are Transfusions Overrated? Surgical Outcome of Jehovah's Witnesses" (1993) 94 Amer. J. of Med.: 118

Koop, C. "The Sanctity of Life" (1978) 75 J. of the Med. Soc. of N. J.: 62

Kouri, R. "Blood Transfusions, Jehovah's Witnesses and the Rule of the Inviolability of the Human Body" (1975) 5 R.D.U.S.: 156

Kreidie, A. "Bloodless Surgery Making a Comeback With Patients" Medical Post (19 October 1993): 19

Kuhse, H., & al. "The Quality/Quantity-of-life Distinction and its Moral Importance for Nurses" (1989) 26 Int. J. Nurs. Stud.: 205

Lammers, P. "Dealing With Other Cultures and Religions Emphasized at Recent Ethics Conference" (1987) 45 AORN J.: 1211

Lehmann "Decision Analysis: A Language for Survival in the Era of Managed Care" (August 1997) Contemp. Ped.: 69

Lindeboom, F. A. "The Story of a Blood Transfusion to a Pope" (1954) 9 J. Hist. Med.: 455

Linden, L. "Living Wills and Substitute Decision-Making" (July 1991) Ont. Med. Rev.: 33

Lloyd, A., & al. "Patients' Ability to Recall Risk Associated With Treatment Options" (1999) 353 The Lancet: 645

MacKenzie, D. "How Safe is Europe's Blood?" (15 January 1994) New Sci.: 12

Macklin, R. "Ethical Relativism in a Multicultural Society" (1998) 8 Kennedy Institute of Ethics J.: 1

Macklin, R. "The Inner Workings of an Ethics Committee: Latest Battle Over Jehovah's Witnesses" (February-March 1988) Hast. Cent. Rep.: 16

Madigan, K. "Presumptions Respecting Mental Competence" (1994) 39 Can. J. Psych. 147

Malyon, D. "Transfusion-Free Treatment of Jehovah's Witnesses: Respecting the Autonomous Patient's Rights" (1998) 24 J. of Med. Ethics: 302

Malyon, D. "Transfusion-Free Treatment of Jehovah's Witnesses: Respecting the Autonomous Patient's Motives" (1998) 24 J. of Med. Ethics: 376

Manners, S. "When Religious Faith Dictates Treatment" (1984) Dec. Canadian Doctor 16

McClintock and Strong's Cyclopoedia, vol. 1 (Grand Rapids: Baker Book House, 1981): 834

McClure, R.D., & Dunn, G.R. "Transfusion of Blood" (March 1917) XXVIII:313 J. H. Hosp. Bull.: 102

Meyers, C. "The Impact of Physician Denial Upon Patient Autonomy and Well-Being" (1992) 18:3 J. Med. Ethics: 135

Minuck, M. & Lambie, R. S. "Anesthesia and Surgery for Jehovah's Witnesses" (27 May 1961) 84 Can. Med. A. J.: 1187

Muramoto, O. "Bioethics of the Refusal of Blood by Jehovah's Witnesses: Part 1. Should Bioethical Deliberation Consider Dissident's Views?" (1998) 24 J. of Med. Ethics: 230

Muramoto, O. "Bioethics of the Refusal of Blood by Jehovah's Witnesses: Part 2. A Novel Approach Based on Rational Non-Interventional Paternalism" (1998) 24 J. of Med. Ethics: 301

Najand, A. "Anesthésiste-réanimateur et Témoins de Jéhovah" (1992) no. 11 Ann. Fr. Anesth. Réanim.: 237

Napier, J. A. "Towards More Rational Use of Red Cells" (1994) 343 The Lancet: 1280

Nau, J.-Y., & Nouchi, F. "Fatal Attraction in Prisoners' Blood" (26 April 1992) Guard. Week.: 15

Nelson, C. L., & al. "Total Hip Arthroplasty in Jehovah's Witnesses without Blood Transfusion" (March 1986) 68-A:3 J. of Bo. & Jt. Surg.: 350

"New Scandal Erupts in France Over Export of Blood Products" The Medical Post (17 November 1992): 60

Nielsen, W. "The Biblical Laws Against Transfusions Reexamined – A Christian Physician's Viewpoint" (October 1991) V:4: 273

Nora, L. "Medicolegal Aspects of Informed Consent" (1998) 16 Neuro. Clin.: 214

Ottenberg, R., & Kaliski, D. J. "Accidents in Transfusion" (13 December 1913) 61 JAMA: 2138

Overs, M. "Patients can refuse treatment by MD" (15 December 1990) Fam. Prac.: 8

Packard, F. R. "Guy Patin and the Medical Profession in Paris in The Seventeenth Century" (1922) IV Ann. of Med. Hist.: 358

Patel, T. "French 'cut corner' Over HIV Testing" (13 March 1993) New Sci.: 13

Pepper, W. "Benjamin Rush" (1890) XIV:17 JAMA: 599

Picard, A. "Blood Victims May See Cash by Year's End" The Globe and Mail (29 November 1993)

Picard, A. "France Makes an Example of Misdeeds" The Globe and Mail (17 September 1993): 219

Picard, A. "Krever report fallout looks devastating" The Globe and Mail (28 November 1997): A1

Picard, A. "Tragedy Prompts Bloodless Solutions" The Globe and Mail (18 May 1996): A1

Picard, E. "Consent to Medical Treatment in Canada" (1981) 19 Osgoode. Hall L. J.: 140

Polk, H., & al. "Blood Management Practice Guidelines: Conference Highlights" (1995) 170 Amer. J. of Surg.: 15

"Prison Sentences for French Blood Transfusion Officials" New Scientist (31 October 1992): 8

Quill, T., & al. "Physician Recommendations and Patient Autonomy: Finding a Balance Between Physician and Patient Choice" (1996) 125 Ann. of Intern. Med.: 764

Rafuse, J. "Better Planning Could Have Saved Life of Woman Who Refused Transfusion, MD says" (1 May 1993) Can. Med. Assoc. J.: 1596

Rhoden "Litigating Life and Death" (1988) 102 Harv. L. Rev.: 375

Ridley, D. "Honoring Jehovah's Witnesses' Advance Directives in Emergencies: A Response to Drs Migden and Braen" (1998) 5 Acad. Emer. Med.: 825

Risse, G. "The Renaissance of Bloodletting: a Chapter in Modern Therapeutics" (1979) 34:1 J. of Med. Hist. Of Med.: 3

Robb, N. "Jehovah's Witnesses Leading Education Drive as Hospitals Adjust to no Blood Requests" (15 February 1996) 154:4 Can. Med. Assoc. J.: 557

Robblee, J.A. "Alternatives to Blood Transfusion: The Surgical Perspective" (Report of proceedings and recommendations of conference Building a Blood System in the 21st Century, Toronto, 3-4 November 1997): 17

Rosam, E. "Patients' Rights and the Role of the Emergency Physician in the Management of Jehovah's Witnesses" (1991) 20 Ann. of Emerg. Med.: 1151

Rothenberg, D. M. "The Approach to the Jehovah's Witness Patient" (1990) 8:3 Anesthesiol. Clin. Of N. Amer.: 589

Routh, C. "Remarks Statistical and General on Transfusion of Blood" (1849) 20 Med. Times: 114

Rozovsky, L., & al. "Jehovah's Witness Case Sets Precedent – Controversy Over a Patient's Right to Refuse Treatment" (May 1990) Physic. Man.: 68

Saéz-Alquézar & al. "Evaluation of the Performance of Brazilian Blood Banks in Testing for Chagas' Disease" (1998) 74 Vox Sanguinis: 228

Sandiford, F. M., & al. "Aorto-Coronary Bypass in Jehovah's Witnesses" (1974) 68 J. of Thor. & Cardio. Surg.: 1

Saxena, S. "Iron-Deficiency Anemia: A Medically Treataable Chronic Anemia as a Model for Transfusion Overuse" (1993) 94 Amerc. J. Of Med.: 121

Sazama, K. "Practical Issues in Informed Consent for Transfusion" (1997) 107 Am. J. Clin. Pathol.: S72

Schmidt, P. J. "Transfusion in America in the Eighteenth and Nineteenth Centuries" 279:24 New Eng. J. of Med.: 1319

Seigworth, G. R. "Bloodletting Over the Centuries" (December 1980) N. Y. St. J. of Med.: 2024

Sevensky, R. "The Religious Foundations of Health-care: A Conceptual Approach" (1983) 9 J. of Med. Ethics: 165

Sher, G. "The Blood Conservation Program at The Toronto Hospital" (Report of proceedings and recommendations of conference for Building a Blood System in the 21st Century, Toronto, 3-4 November 1997): 46

Siddall, A.C. "Bloodletting in American Obstetric Practice, 1800-1945" (1980) 54 Bull. of the Hist. of Med.: 102

Spence R. K., et al. "Elective Surgery without Transfusion: Influence of Preoperative Hemoglobin Level and Blood Loss on Mortality" (1990) 159 Am. J. of Surg.: 320

Spence, R. K., & al. "Transfusion and Surgery" (1993) XXX Curr. Prob. In Surg.: 1105

Spence, R. K. "The Effects of Hemoglobin Levels and Blood Loss on Surgical Mortality" (July 1989) Inf. Surg.: 264

Spence, R. K. "The Status of Bloodless Surgery" (1991) V Transf. Med. Rev.: 274

Spence, R. "Blood Management Policies for Jehovah's Witnesses" Appendix 2 (1995) 170 Amer. J. of Surg.: 148

Stehling & al. "A Survey of Transfusion Practices Among Anesthesiologists" (1987) 52 Vos Sanguinis: 61

Stevenson, M. "Refusing Measles Vaccine May Put Others at Risk: Study" The Gazette (7 July 1999): A12

Tartter, P. I. "Immunologic Effects of Blood Transfusions" (1995) 24 Immuno Inv.: 277

The College of Physicians and Surgeons of Ontario, College Notices, Issue No. 21, Nov. 1990

Thomas, J. E. "Ethical Reflections on Patient Refusals of Life-Saving Treatment" (1991) 5:4 Transf. Med. Rev.: 259

Thomas, J. M. "Nonblood Management in Obstetrics and Gynaecology" (May 1997) J. SOGC: 475

Thomson & al. "Blood Component Treatment: A Retrospective Audit in Five Major London Hospitals" (1991) no. 44 Clin. Path.: 734

Trent, B. "Jehovah's Witnesses and the Transfusion Debate: "We are not Asking for the Right to Die" (1991) 114:770 Can. Med. Assoc. J.: 774

Two Hospitals Offering Patients Options of "Bloodless Surgery" 13:12 Mod. Health: 50

U.S Congress, Office of Technology Assessment Task Force, Blood Technologies, Services, and Issues (1988): 121

Unger "Medical-Legal Aspects of Blood Transfusion" (1960) 60:2 N. Y. St. J. of Med.: 237

Viele, M., & al. "What can we Learn About the Need for Transfusion from Patients who Refuse Blood" (1994) 34 Transf.: 396

Wahi, J. "Are Living Wills Valid?" (May-June 1990) Home Health-care: 38

Williamson, L., & al. "Reporting Serious Hazards of Transfusions: The SHOT Program" (1998) 12 Trans. Med. Rev.: 28

Winslow, R., professor of Medicine at the University of California at San Diego during the presentation "Is There A Potential Need for Blood Substitutes in Civilian and Noncivilian Situations?" (Address to the IV International Symposium on Blood Substitutes, 20 August 1991)

Wreen, M. "Autonomy, Religious Values, and Refusal of Lifesaving Medical T-eatment" (1991) 17 J. Med. Ethics: 124

Zauder, H. L. "How Did We Get a "Magic Number" for Preoperative Hematocrit/Hemoglobin Level?" (Address to the National institutes of Health Consensus Development Conference, 27 June 1988)

Zeitz, E. "Legal Reasoning and Medical Decision Making" (1998) 5 Acad. Emerg. Med.: 755

INDEX

A

B

C

K

L

M

N

O

P

Q

R

S

T

U

V

W

STUDIES IN RELIGION AND SOCIETY

1. Anson D. Shupe, **Six Perpsectives on New Religions: A Case Study Approach**
2. Barry Cooper, **Michel Foucault: An Introduction to the Study of His Thought**
3. Eileen Barker (ed.), **New Religious Movements: A Perspective for Understanding Society**
4. Christine Elizabeth King, **The Nazi State and the New Religions: Five Case Studies in Non-Conformity**
5. David G. Bromley and James T. Richardson (eds.), **The Brainwashing/Deprogramming Controversy: Sociological, Psychological, Legal and Historical Perspectives**
6. Tom Craig Darrand and Anson Shupe, **Metaphors of Social Control in a Pentecostal Sect**
7. Judith Mary Weightman, **Making Sense of the Jonestown Suicides: A Sociological History of the Peoples Temple**
8. Barbara Hargrove (ed.), **Religion and the Sociology of Knowledge: Modernization and Pluralism in Christian Thought and Structure**
9. Niklas Luhmann, **Religious Dogmatics and the Evolution of Societies**, introduction by Peter Beyer (trans.)
10. Herbert Richardson (ed.), **Constitutional Issues in the Case of Reverend Moon: *Amicus* Briefs Presented to the United States Supreme Court**
11. Annette P. Hampshire, **Mormonism in Conflict: The Nauvoo Years**
12. Patricia Werhane and Kendall D'Andrade (eds.), **Profit and Responsibility: Issues in Business and Professional Ethics**
13. James H. Grace, **Sex and Marriage in the Unification Movement: A Sociological Study**
14. Rebecca Moore, **A Sympathetic History of Jonestown: The Moore Family Involvement in Peoples Temple**
15. Tommy H. Poling and J. Frank Kenney, **The Hare Krishna Character Type: A Study of the Sensate Personality**
16. Edward C. Lehman, Jr., **Women Clergy in England: Sexism, Modern Consciousness, and Church Viability**
17. Joseph H. Fichter, **Autobiographies of Conversion**
18. George B. Pepper, **The Boston Heresy Case in View of the Secularization of Religion: A Case Study in the Sociology of Religion**
19. Leo Driedger, **Mennonite Identity in Conflict**
20. Helen Ralston, **Christian Ashrams: A New Religious Movement in Contemporary India**
21. Martha F. Lee, **The Nation of Islam, An American Millennarian Movement**
22. James T. Richardson (ed.), **Money and Power in the New Religions**
23. Sharon Linzey Georgianna, **The Moral Majority and Fundamentalism: Plausibility and Dissonance**

24. Roger O'Toole (ed.), **Sociological Studies in Roman Catholicism: Historical and Contemporary Perspectives**

25. Frank D. Schubert, **A Sociological Study of Secularization Trends in the American Catholic University: Decatholicizing the Catholic Religious Curriculum**

26. Hal W. French, **A Study of Religious Fanaticism and Responses To It: Adversary Identity**

27. A.D. Wright, **Catholicism and Spanish Society Under the Reign of Philip II, 1555-1598, and Philip III, 1598-1621**

28. Theodore Weinberger, **Strategies for Sustaining Religious Commitment: The Art of the Religious Life**

29. George W. Buchanan, **Biblical and Theological Insights from Ancient and Modern Civil Law**

30. James Thrower, **Marxism-Leninism as the Civil Religion of Soviet Society: God's Commissar**

31. Phebe Davidson (ed.), **New Readings of Spiritual Narrative From the Fifteenth to the Twentieth Century: Secular Force and Self-Disclosure**

32. Radu Dragan and Augustin Ioan, **Symbols and Language in Sacred Christian Architecture**

33. George B. von der Lippe, **The Figure of Martin Luther in Twentieth-Century German Literature: The Metamorphosis of a National Symbol**

34. Pink Dandelion, **A Sociological Analysis of the Theology of Quakers: The Silent Revolution**

35. Kjell Nordstokke, **Council and Context in Leonardo Boff's Ecclesiology: The Rebirth of the Church Among the Poor**, translated from the Norwegian by Brian MacNeil

36. John W. Lynes, **Themes in the Current Reformation in Religious Thinking**

37. Vasil Gluchman, **Slovak Lutheran Social Ethics**

38. Robert H. Ayers, **Christian Theology in a Contemporary World**

39. James T. Bretzke, S.J. (compiler), **Bibliography on Scripture and Christian Ethics**

40. Malcolm R. Thorp, **Herbert Butterfield and the Reinterpretation of the Christian Historical Perspective**

41. John W. Kleiner (ed.), **Henry Melchior Muhlenberg– The Roots of 250 Years of Organized Lutheranism in North America: Essays in Memory of Helmut T. Lehmann**

42. Thomas J. Scirghi, **An Examination of the Problems of Inclusive Language in the Trinitarian Formula of Baptism**

43. J. Kevin Coyle and Steven C. Muir (eds.), **Healing in Religion and Society, From Hippocrates to the Puritans: Selected Studies**

44. Stewart A. Dippel, **The Professionalization of the English Church From 1560 to 1700: Ambassadors for Christ**

45. Brett Knowles, **The History of a New Zealand Pentecostal Movement: The New Life Churches of New Zealand From 1946 to 1979**

46. Rupe Simms, **The Politics of Accommodation and Resistance in the Black Church: A Gramscian Analysis**
47. Theodore Gabriel, **Hindu and Muslim Inter-Religious Relations in Malaysia**
48. David A. Copeland, **Benjamin Keach and the Development of Baptist Traditions in Seventeenth-Century England**
49. Okbazghi Yohannes, **Political Economy of an Authoritarian Modern State and Religious Nationalism in Egypt**
50. Brian E. Strayer, **Huguenots and Camisards as Aliens in France, 1598-1789: The Struggle for Religious Toleration**
51. Michael J. McGrath, **Religious Celebrations in Segovia, 1577-1697**
52. Nickolas K. Gvosdev, **An Examination of Church-State Relations in the Byzantine and Russian Empires with an Emphasis on Ideology and Models of Interaction**
53. Hilmi M. Zawati, **Is Jihād a Just War? War, Peace, and Human Rights Under Islamic and Public International Law**
54. Andrew D. Penny, **John Foxe, Evangelicalism, and the Oxford Movement: Dialogue Across the Centuries**
55. Julian Jenkins, **Christian Pacifism Confronts German Nationalism–The Ecumenical Movement and the Cause of Peace in Germany, 1914-1933**
56. Anthony J. Blasi and Bernard F. Donahoe, **A History of Sociological Research and Teaching at Catholic Notre Dame University, Indiana**
57. Daniel Capper, **Guru Devotion and the American Buddhist Experience**
58. Ina Merdjanova, **Religion, Nationalism, and Civil Society in Eastern Europe–The Postcommunist Palimpsest**
59. Cyril G. Williams (ed.), **Contemporary Conceptions of God–Interdisciplinary Essays**
60. Martin L. Warren, **Asceticism in the Christian Transformation of Self in Margery Kempe, William Thorpe, and John Rogers**
61. Santosh C. Saha and Thomas K. Carr (eds.), **Islamic, Hindu, and Christian Fundamentalism Compared–Public Policy in Global Perspective**
62. Malcolm Gold, **The Hybridization of an Assembly of God Church–Proselytism, Retention, and Re-Affiliation**
63. André Carbonneau, **Ethical Issues and the Religious and Historical Basis for the Objection of Jehovah's Witnesses to Blood Transfusion Therapy**
64. E. James Baesler, **Theoretical Explorations and Empirical Investigations of Communication and Prayer**